FAST FACTS

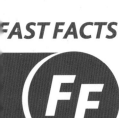

W9-BGJ-306

Hyperlipidemia

ndispensable
Guides to
Clinical
Practice

Second edition

Paul Durrington
Professor of Medicine,
University of Manchester,
Department of Medicine,
Manchester Royal Infirmary, UK

Allan Sniderman
Edwards Professor of Cardiology
and Professor of Medicine,
McGill University, Montreal, Canada

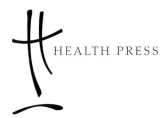

HEALTH PRESS

Oxford

Fast Facts – Hyperlipidemia
First published 2000
Second edition November 2002

Text © 2002 Paul Durrington, Allan Sniderman
© in this edition Health Press 2002
Health Press Limited, Elizabeth House, Queen Street, Abingdon,
Oxford OX14 3JR, UK
Tel: +44 (0)1235 523233
Fax: +44 (0)1235 523238

Fast Facts is a trade mark of Health Press Limited.

The publisher and the authors have made every effort to ensure the
accuracy of this book, but cannot accept responsibility for any errors
or omissions.

The authors are indebted to Caroline Price for her expert preparation
of the original manuscript and to the University of Manchester
Department of Medical Illustration, UK, for many of the figures. We
also gratefully acknowledge the great support of colleagues,
particularly Paul Miller. This book is dedicated to our wives.

A CIP catalogue record for this title is available from the British
Library.

ISBN 1-903734-23-1

Durrington, P (Paul)
Fast Facts – Hyperlipidemia/
Paul Durrington, Allan Sniderman

Illustrated by MeDee Art, London, UK.

Typesetting and page layout by Zed, Oxford, UK.

Printed by Fine Print (Services) Ltd, Oxford, UK.

Glossary

Android obesity: male-pattern obesity, characterized by increased accumulation of abdominal adipose tissue

Apob$_{100}$: hepatic apolipoprotein B

Apob$_{48}$: gut apolipoprotein B (its molecular weight is 48% of that of apob$_{100}$)

Apolipoproteins: structural proteins, often containing receptor binding sites

ASP: acylation-stimulating protein

ATPIII: Third Adult Treatment Panel of the NCEP

β-VLDL: chylomicron remnants and intermediate-density lipoprotein

CE: cholesteryl ester

CETP: cholesteryl ester transfer protein, which catalyzes transfer of cholesterol from HDL to circulating triglyceride-rich lipoproteins, and from LDL back to VLDL

CHD: coronary heart disease

Cholesteryl ester: esterified cholesterol, which is more hydrophobic than free cholesterol

FC: free cholesterol

FFA: free fatty acids

FH: familial hypercholesterolemia

Foam cell: a cell, usually a macrophage, the cytoplasm of which has become loaded with cholesterol

Gynoid obesity: female-pattern obesity, characterized by increased depots in the buttocks and other peripheral sites

HDL: high-density lipoprotein

IDL: intermediate-density lipoprotein

LCAT: lecithin–cholesterol acyl transferase, which catalyzes the esterification of free cholesterol

LDL: low-density lipoprotein

Lipemia retinalis: pallor of the optic fundus and white appearance of the retinal veins and arteries due to extremely high levels of circulating chylomicrons

Lp(a): lipoprotein (a), an LDL-like particle that contains apolipoprotein (a) in addition to apob

LPL: lipoprotein lipase, an enzyme which breaks down triglycerides into fatty acids

LpX: lipoprotein X, an abnormal lipoprotein present in plasma in obstructive jaundice

NCEP: National Cholesterol Education Program

NEFA: non-esterified fatty acids

Small, dense LDL: cholesterol-depleted LDL that is not cleared through the LDL receptors, and is more atherogenic than normal LDL because it is readily oxidized

VLDL: very-low-density lipoprotein

A note on conversion of units

So that values will accord more closely with those chosen by various consensus groups, we have used a factor of 40, rather than the more precise 38.6, to convert between mmol/L and mg/dL as units of cholesterol concentration. Similarly, a conversion factor of 90 has been used for triglycerides. Converted values are given to two significant figures.

Introduction

This second edition is directed at a broad range of healthcare professionals, from family physicians to specialists. Our objective is to present a crisp and accurate summary of the field. In particular, we wanted to outline a coherent pathophysiologic structure on which the physician can build a sound diagnostic and clinical approach.

Vascular disease is not beaten, but it is retreating, and it is therefore critical that we apply as rapidly as possible the major clinical and scientific advances that have occurred. Guidelines are one way to speed implementation – they are invaluable for guiding clinical practice – but they do not substitute for clear knowledge of the issues at stake.

As physicians, we need to know not only what to do, but also why we need to do it. We need not only to understand what the evidence supports today, but to have the knowledge that will allow us to understand the advances that are going to be presented tomorrow. We need to know not only what is right in general, but how to craft the best treatment for the patient in front of us right now.

In that spirit, we make no apology for providing a text that interprets clinical trial evidence in the context of pathogenesis and gives practical solutions to routine problems encountered in the clinical management of hyperlipidemias.

Our objective in this book is to present an up-to-date review of the diagnosis and therapy of the common atherogenic dyslipoproteinemias. This means we will try to show the reader both where practice stands now and where it is going.

For example, clinical practice has traditionally been based on the serum concentration of cholesterol and triglycerides in plasma as well as on that of cholesterol contained in low-density and high-density lipoprotein (LDL and HDL, respectively) particles. Among all these, LDL cholesterol has been declared the most important. To assess accurately the risk from LDL, however, one needs to know not only the amount of LDL cholesterol but also the number of LDL particles per deciliter of serum and also the size of the particles (see page 10 and Chapter 2). The amount of cholesterol in lipoprotein particles – particularly in the case of LDL – varies with the size of the particle. Therefore, a knowledge of the LDL cholesterol level is not in itself sufficient to establish accurately the number of LDL particles. Unfortunately, the tools to determine particle number and size are not yet as widely available as they should be. We thus discuss management of hyperlipidemia from the conventional point of view, but also take the opportunity to demonstrate what is added by a knowledge of particle number.

Lipoprotein structure

Lipoprotein particles are macromolecular complexes of lipids – cholesterol, cholesteryl ester, triglycerides and phospholipids – and proteins (Figure 1.1). The outer membrane of all lipoprotein particles is made up of a monolayer of phospholipids. Phospholipids are the most highly charged of the lipids because of the phosphate group they contain at one end. At the other end are the long hydrocarbon sequences of the fatty acyl groups, which are not water soluble. Thus, one end of the phospholipid molecule is oriented towards water whereas the other seeks non-polar substances such as lipids. This is why

7

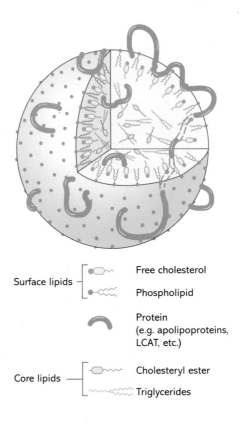

Surface lipids
- Free cholesterol
- Phospholipid

Protein
(e.g. apolipoproteins,
LCAT, etc.)

Core lipids
- Cholesteryl ester
- Triglycerides

Figure 1.1 The structure of a lipoprotein. The most hydrophobic components (the triglycerides and cholesteryl esters) form a central droplet, which is surrounded by the more polar components (free cholesterol, proteins and phospholipids). Proteins are arranged with their hydrophobic sequences inside the particle, whereas their hydrophilic regions are oriented towards the aqueous environment. The polar groups of cholesterol and phospholipids also point outwards, away from the hydrophobic core.

phospholipids are ideal materials to encase the core lipids – triglycerides and cholesteryl ester – so these insoluble lipids can be transported in plasma.

Apolipoproteins are proteins found in the phospholipid external monolayer of the lipoproteins. They differ in function and in whether or not they can leave one particle for another. Each very-low-density lipoprotein (VLDL) and LDL particle contains one molecule of the B apolipoprotein apoB$_{100}$, whereas each chylomicron particle contains one molecule of a truncated version of apoB$_{100}$, called apoB$_{48}$. Both apoB$_{100}$ and apoB$_{48}$ remain with their respective particles until they are removed from the circulation. Not only does apoB$_{100}$ provide structural integrity to the particle, but also a critical region binds to the LDL receptor, and it is this interaction which results in the irreversible removal of LDL from plasma.

ApoB-positive particles are atherogenic. Because there is one apoB molecule per particle, plasma apoB level gives an exact measure of the number of apoB-positive particles; further, because chylomicron particles never constitute more than 1% and VLDL particles account for less than 10% of lipoprotein particles, the level of apoB gives a good estimate of LDL particle number. Chylomicrons are few in number even postprandially, so patients do not have to be fasting when plasma apoB level is measured.

The four types of lipoprotein particle

Chylomicrons and VLDL are the two triglyceride-rich lipoproteins whereas LDL and HDL are the two cholesterol-rich lipoproteins. All four are illustrated in Figure 1.2.

Chylomicrons and VLDL. Chylomicrons are much larger than VLDL and correspondingly contain much more triglyceride per particle. Both chylomicrons and VLDL contain several other apolipoproteins on their surface. Among these are the C apolipoproteins, of which apoCII and apoCIII regulate the rate at which triglyceride hydrolysis occurs. ApoCII is an essential cofactor for lipoprotein lipase, the enzyme which breaks down the triglyceride, whereas apoCIII, at least in excess, delays triglyceride clearance, although the mechanisms by which this occurs are not entirely clear. ApoE is also present on the surface of chylomicrons and VLDL, and it plays an important role in regulating the rate at which their remnants are removed by the liver. ApoAI and apoAII are also present and transfer back and forth to HDL particles.

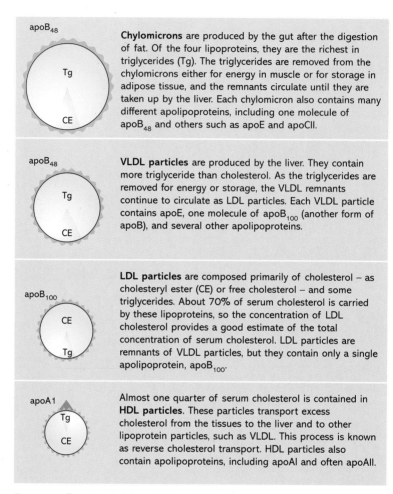

apoB₄₈

Chylomicrons are produced by the gut after the digestion of fat. Of the four lipoproteins, they are the richest in triglycerides (Tg). The triglycerides are removed from the chylomicrons either for energy in muscle or for storage in adipose tissue, and the remnants circulate until they are taken up by the liver. Each chylomicron also contains many different apolipoproteins, including one molecule of apoB₄₈ and others such as apoE and apoCII.

apoB₄₈

VLDL particles are produced by the liver. They contain more triglyceride than cholesterol. As the triglycerides are removed for energy or storage, the VLDL remnants continue to circulate as LDL particles. Each VLDL particle contains apoE, one molecule of apoB₁₀₀ (another form of apoB), and several other apolipoproteins.

apoB₁₀₀

LDL particles are composed primarily of cholesterol – as cholesteryl ester (CE) or free cholesterol – and some triglycerides. About 70% of serum cholesterol is carried by these lipoproteins, so the concentration of LDL cholesterol provides a good estimate of the total concentration of serum cholesterol. LDL particles are remnants of VLDL particles, but they contain only a single apolipoprotein, apoB₁₀₀.

apoA1

Almost one quarter of serum cholesterol is contained in **HDL particles**. These particles transport excess cholesterol from the tissues to the liver and to other lipoprotein particles, such as VLDL. This process is known as reverse cholesterol transport. HDL particles also contain apolipoproteins, including apoAI and often apoAII.

Figure 1.2 Four types of lipoprotein particle.

LDL. Most of the cholesterol present in plasma is found in LDL particles. LDL particles, however, vary in size with the amount of cholesterol they contain (Figure 1.3). The smaller particles contain less cholesterol and, since lipids are less dense than proteins, are therefore denser than the larger particles. This is a very important distinction because, particle for particle, smaller, denser LDL are more atherogenic than larger, more buoyant LDL.

The process by which small, dense LDL particles are formed is illustrated in Figure 1.4. Step 1 occurs when cholesteryl ester transfer

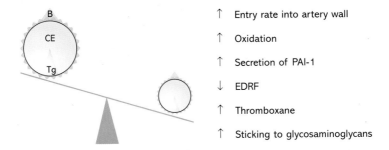

	↑ Entry rate into artery wall
	↑ Oxidation
	↑ Secretion of PAI-1
	↓ EDRF
	↑ Thromboxane
	↑ Sticking to glycosaminoglycans

Figure 1.3 Why small, dense LDL particles are more atherogenic than normal, larger LDL. CE, cholesteryl ester; Tg, triglyceride; PAI-1, plasminogen activator inhibitor type 1; EDRF, endothelium-derived relaxing factor.

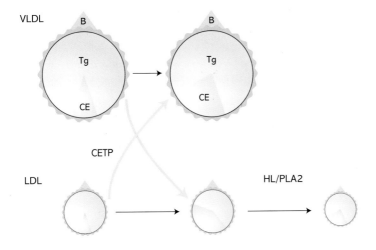

Figure 1.4 How small, dense LDL are formed in plasma: LDL remodeling by cholesterol–triglyceride exchange and hydrolysis. CETP, cholesteryl ester transfer protein; HL, hepatic lipase; PLA2, phospholipase A2.

protein (CETP) allows a cholesteryl ester molecule from an LDL particle to be exchanged for a triglyceride molecule from VLDL. Step 2 occurs when the triglyceride is hydrolyzed either by hepatic lipase or by another enzyme such as phospholipase A2 to produce a smaller, denser LDL particle.

11

HDL plays a critical role in the transport of cholesterol from peripheral cells to the liver. Low levels of HDL are associated with an increased risk of coronary heart disease (CHD), a relation which is particularly prominent when LDL levels – either LDL cholesterol or apoB concentration – are elevated. HDL levels are generally low in patients with hypertriglyceridemia by virtue of the same remodeling mechanisms that are responsible for the generation of small, dense LDL particles. HDL levels can be quantified either by measuring HDL cholesterol or by measuring the level of the major apolipoprotein in HDL: apoAI. Unfortunately, there is no direct relation between apoAI level and HDL particle number. Nevertheless, there is now evidence that plasma levels of apoAI are at least as informative of cardiovascular risk as levels of HDL cholesterol.

How do lipoprotein particles transport lipids?

Lipoproteins transport triglycerides and cholesterol from one point in the body to another. In this section, we briefly review first the transport of fatty acids, whether bound to plasma (non-esterified fatty acids, NEFA) or within triglycerides, and then turn to the transport of cholesterol.

Triglyceride transport and storage. Triglycerides are an almost ideal form of energy storage and consequently are, far and away, the major form in which we store energy. Almost one fifth of the total mass of a lean 70 kg adult man is made up of triglyceride in adipose tissue. If oxidized, this would yield 570 000 kilojoules – roughly enough energy to survive total starvation for 3 months. Certainly in the long term, triglycerides are a far more important source of energy than glycogen, the total store of which would yield fewer than 4200 kilojoules.

Adipose tissue is the major site of triglyceride storage, and the adipose cell appears morphologically to be no more than a rim of cytoplasm around a large central droplet of triglyceride. These cells, however, are much more active metabolically than their structure suggests. Not only is the rate at which they take up and release fatty acids tightly regulated, but they also synthesize and secrete a wide variety of bioactive molecules, some of which, such as acylation stimulating protein (ASP), appear to play critical roles in their handling of fatty acids. Insulin also plays a critical role in regulating fatty acid uptake and release.

The metabolism of chylomicrons and VLDL is illustrated in Figure 1.5. Dietary triglycerides undergo digestion in the gut to fatty acids and monoglycerides. These are absorbed into the enterocytes, resynthesized into triglycerides and packaged into chylomicrons, and then enter the circulation for transport to the tissues. Fat absorption is generally complete within a few hours, and during this time plasma triglyceride levels increase, although the degree to which they do is very modest in healthy people. In some people, however, their clearance is delayed and postprandial hypertriglyceridemia is an important clinical finding.

At the capillary endothelial surfaces in adipose tissue and in cardiac and skeletal muscle, the enzyme lipoprotein lipase (LPL) rapidly breaks down the triglycerides within chylomicrons, releasing large amounts of fatty acids. Muscle is extremely effective at taking up these fatty acids, most of which are almost immediately oxidized for energy. Surprisingly, adipose tissue is less effective, with only about two thirds of the fatty acids which were released being taken up on average; the rest are bound to albumin and then circulate in plasma as NEFA.

After encountering LPL, chylomicrons become relatively triglyceride-poor and cholesterol-rich remnants. Normally, these chylomicron remnants are rapidly removed by the liver. This is fortunate because, if they accumulate in plasma, they are extremely atherogenic (see Chapter 6, Type III hyperlipoproteinemia).

The fatty acids taken up by adipocytes are reformed into triglycerides. During fasting, when energy is required elsewhere, the adipose tissue triglycerides are hydrolyzed by an intracellular enzyme, hormone-sensitive lipase, releasing fatty acids from adipose tissue. When large amounts of energy are required rapidly, as during exercise, the activity of hormone-sensitive lipase is increased by catecholamines, releasing additional fatty acids as metabolic fuel.

VLDL particles undergo the same metabolic fate as chylomicrons, with one important difference. Just as with chylomicrons, the triglyceride within them is broken down by LPL on the capillary

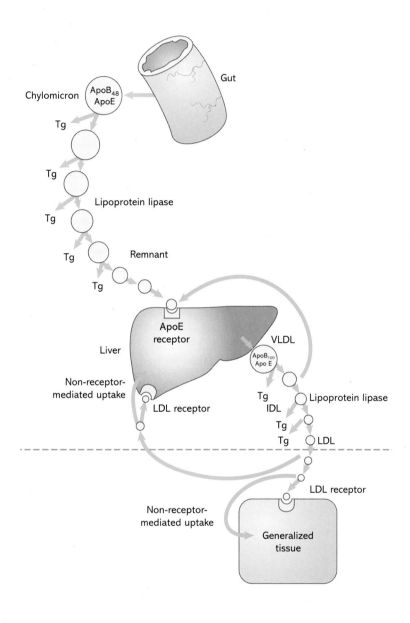

Figure 1.5 Metabolism of chylomicrons, VLDL and LDL. Tg, triglyceride; IDL, intermediate-density lipoprotein.

endothelium of muscle and adipose tissue, and fatty acids are released which may be taken up by adipose tissue or muscle or circulate as NEFA. However, whereas the chylomicron remnants produced are, in general, rapidly removed from the circulation by the liver, most VLDL particles become converted to LDL particles.

LDL particles persist in plasma nine times longer than VLDL particles. That is why there are always nine times more LDL than VLDL particles. In addition, LDL particles are much smaller than VLDL particles. Those two facts explain why LDL is more directly important in atherogenesis than VLDL.

Another point to note is that the proportion of fatty acids taken up by adipose tissue, as opposed to the proportion persisting in the circulation, is variable. This is due in part to variation in the efficiency of the mechanism for trapping fatty acids in the adipose tissue. If fewer fatty acids are taken up by adipose tissue, more remain in the circulation, with the result that there is an increased flux of fatty acids to the liver, where they are synthesized into triglycerides and released as VLDL. This will result in much greater secretion of VLDL particles into plasma. If the number released is in excess of oxidative needs, this also results in increased flux of fatty acids to the liver and increased formation of VLDL and then LDL particles.

Fatty acid trapping is therefore a critical process, and we are only beginning to understand its pathophysiological determinants. Insulin and acylation-stimulating protein (ASP) are the two for which most direct evidence has been found. ASP is a breakdown product of the interaction of three proteins secreted by adipocytes: the third component of complement (C3), adipsin and Factor B. It is not widely appreciated that adipose tissue is a very active metabolic organ which produces a wide range of bioactive molecules – leptin and ASP being only two examples.

Both ASP and insulin increase the rate at which fatty acids are formed into triglycerides by adipocytes, and reduce the rate at which they are released from them. Importantly, their effects are independent and additive. Both therefore increase fatty acid trapping. If insulin resistance or ASP resistance occur, the effectiveness of fatty acid trapping is reduced and fatty acid flux to the liver and skeletal muscle increases, resulting in dyslipidemia (hyperTg, hyperapoB) and dysglycemia (hyperinsulinemia or type 2 diabetes mellitus); see Chapter 7.

Cholesterol metabolism and transport in lipoproteins. Typically, the daily cholesterol intake is 200–500 mg/day, whereas total dietary fat intake is 80–100 g/day. Furthermore, cholesterol absorption from the gut is incomplete, with only 30–60% actually entering the body. All the cells in the body can synthesize cholesterol, and taken together the body synthesizes at least as much cholesterol as it absorbs.

The ability to synthesize cholesterol is vital, as it is an essential component of cell membranes and the precursor of steroid hormones and vitamin D. Almost all tissues can synthesize cholesterol, although most synthesis is centralized to the liver, the gut and the central nervous system. Cholesterol biosynthesis is extremely complex. However, a key regulatory step occurs early in the pathway, at the point where 3-hydroxy-3-methylglutaryl CoA is converted to mevalonic acid. The enzyme responsible, HMG-CoA reductase, can be inhibited by a variety of factors, the most important of which, for clinical purposes, is the class of the statin drugs (otherwise known as HMG-CoA reductase inhibitors).

The liver is the central clearing house for cholesterol, with several ways in and out. Although all the body's cells can synthesize cholesterol, only hepatocytes can break it down to bile acids or secrete cholesterol dissolved in bile acids into the small intestine. This is the major route by which cholesterol can leave the body. Of the total reaching the small intestine, however, a variable but important amount is reabsorbed, resulting in enterohepatic cholesterol cycling. Interruption of this cycle by cholesterol absorption inhibitors, such as plant sterol or stanol esters added to food products, or the drug ezetimibe, lowers serum cholesterol.

Hepatic secretion of cholesterol, mostly as VLDL, exceeds the requirement of tissues. This cholesterol must return to the liver via either LDL or HDL particles if it is not to accumulate in the tissues. However, this is a largely futile and potentially dangerous (atherosclerotic) cycle. Chylomicron remnants transport cholesterol of exogenous origin to the liver.

HDL and reverse cholesterol transport

HDL plays a critical role in the transport of cholesterol from peripheral tissues back to the liver (Figure 1.6). Small HDL particles receive free cholesterol from peripheral tissues, most of which is quickly converted to cholesteryl ester by the enzyme lecithin–cholesterol acyl transferase (LCAT). The cholesteryl ester formed is much more hydrophobic than free cholesterol and so can be tightly packed within the core of the HDL particle, allowing HDL to pick up more cholesterol. Either cholesterol can be returned to the liver directly by an HDL particle or the cholesteryl ester can be transferred by the action of cholesteryl ester

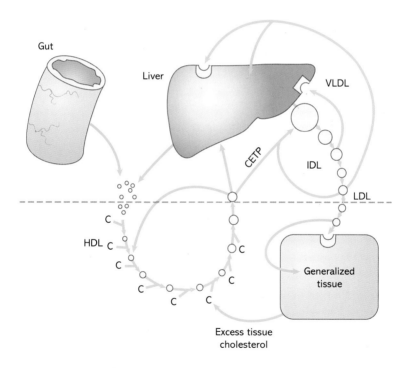

Figure 1.6 HDL is involved in reverse cholesterol transport. Excess cholesterol (C) from the tissues is released to HDL and is then either delivered to the liver or to VLDL in a process mediated by cholesteryl ester transfer protein (CETP). Some cholesteryl ester can be returned to the liver on LDL, but it can also find its way back to the tissues. IDL, intermediate-density lipoprotein.

transfer protein (CETP) in plasma to VLDL in exchange for triglyceride. The cholesteryl ester can then be returned to the liver as VLDL, and/or LDL particles are taken up by it. It can also, of course, be delivered back to the tissues in the same lipoproteins, making CETP potentially atherogenic. Drugs to inhibit CETP are currently undergoing clinical evaluation.

Epidemiological studies have repeatedly shown that the two major determinants of the risk of vascular disease are LDL and HDL. Risk increases as LDL increases. However, at any level of LDL, risk is also determined by HDL. Low levels of HDL are associated with an increased risk of coronary artery disease, and HDL is believed to play a major protective role against atherosclerosis. This could occur in many ways. One is by promoting the transfer of cholesterol from peripheral tissues such as the arterial wall to the liver. Another important mechanism could be by protecting LDL against atherogenic oxidative modification, because the enzyme paraoxonase, located on HDL, can break down lipid peroxides formed on LDL and cell membranes.

Lipids and lipoproteins – structure and physiology – Key points

- LDL particles are the smallest and by far the most numerous of the atherogenic particles. This explains why statin-induced LDL lowering has been so successful in reducing coronary events.
- LDL particles differ in composition, and LDL cholesterol level is therefore often not an accurate guide to LDL particle number.
- The major effect of triglycerides on risk of coronary heart disease is probably due to the production of small, dense LDL particles.
- HDL particles transport cholesterol from the periphery to the liver, although whether this is their only, or even their most important, antiatherogenic effect is not clear.

Key references

Cahill GF. Starvation in man. *N Engl J Med* 1970;282:668–75.

Durrington PN. Lipids and their metabolism. In: *Hyperlipidaemia, Diagnosis and Management,* 2nd edn. Oxford: Butterworth-Heinemann, 1995:4–24.

Durrington PN. Lipoproteins and their metabolism. In: *Hyperlipidaemia, Diagnosis and Management,* 2nd edn. Oxford: Butterworth-Heinemann, 1995:25–71.

Gibbons GF, Mitropoulos K, Myant NB. *Biochemistry of Cholesterol,* 4th edn. Amsterdam: Elsevier, 1982.

Gurr MI, James AT. *Lipid Biochemistry: an Introduction.* London: Chapman and Hall, 1991.

Packard CJ, Shepherd J. Physiology of the lipoprotein transport system: an overview of lipoprotein metabolism. In: Betteridge DJ et al., eds. *Lipoproteins in Health and Disease.* London: Arnold, 1999:17–30.

Sniderman AD, Cianflone K, Arner P et al. The adipocyte, fatty acid trapping, and atherogenesis. *Arterioscler Thromb Vasc Biol* 1998;18:147–51.

Lipids, lipoproteins and the risk of coronary disease

Lipids: cholesterol, triglyceride and HDL cholesterol. The well-known and well-established relationship between the level of cholesterol and the risk of coronary disease is illustrated in Figure 2.1. These data from the MRFIT study demonstrate a curvilinear relation between cholesterol level and risk. Over the whole range, there is a substantial increase in risk. However from the 30th to the 90th percentile of the population, the range which encompasses the vast majority of patients with coronary disease, risk does not increase substantially. Thus, while individuals with very high levels of total and/or LDL cholesterol are at substantially increased risk and those with very low levels are at low risk, most patients with coronary disease have levels of total or LDL cholesterol that are average for their society.

If we define a high cholesterol level as one exceeding the 75th percentile, then low HDL cholesterol (or apoAI) is much more common in coronary patients than high cholesterol. The level of HDL, whether measured as HDL cholesterol or apoAI, is accepted as a major risk factor for coronary disease. Similarly, hypertriglyceridemia is much more common in coronary patients than hypercholesterolemia (usually in combination with low HDL cholesterol).

However, controversy continues in some quarters as to whether triglycerides are really a risk factor for coronary disease. There are several reasons for the persistent debate. First, although a risk factor for vascular disease on univariate analysis, hypertriglyceridemia usually does not remain significant on mulitivariate analysis. However, this may hide the true importance of triglycerides because they are more variable than other risk factors included in multivariate analyses, such as HDL cholesterol, with which they are strongly inversely correlated. This means that they lose out unfairly to HDL cholesterol in such an analysis because of a phenomenon known as regression dilution bias.

Second, CHD is not increased in familial lipoprotein lipase deficiency (see Chapter 5) which gives rise to very high levels of triglycerides. There is a substantially increased risk of pancreatitis rather than coronary disease. This may be because in most patients with very extreme hypertriglyceridemia, LDL levels are low.

Third, the results of the clinical trials of fibrate drugs which predominantly lower serum triglycerides are confusing. In two (BIP and

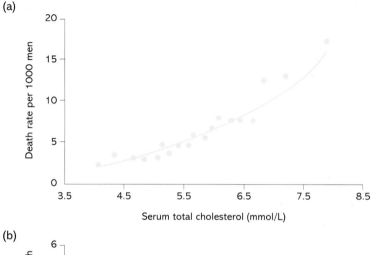

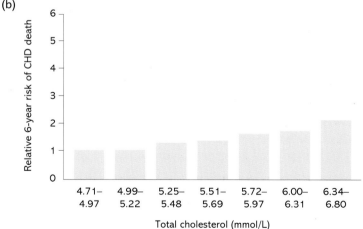

Figure 2.1 (a) Relationship between serum cholesterol levels and CHD mortality in men. Data are from the MRFIT study (La Rosa JC et al. *Circulation* 1990; 81:1721–33). (b) Relative 6-year risk of CHD mortality in the MRFIT study from the 30th to the 90th percentile total cholesterol. Source: Stamler J et al. *JAMA* 1986;256:2823–8.

Helsinki) the decrease in CHD risk was related to the serum triglyceride level whereas in another (VAHIT) it was not. Whether this is another statistical artifact, in this case due to sample size, is not clear. In addition, it must be appreciated that fibrates have additional effects such as raising HDL cholesterol and reducing the number of small, dense LDL particles.

There is no doubt that a greater degree of risk attaches to the LDL cholesterol level when triglycerides are raised and/or HDL is low. This is the important clinical lesson regardless of the precise position of the battle lines of opposing academics.

ApoB and small, dense LDL. The paradoxes concerning triglyceride may be more apparent than real, and most can be resolved by taking into account LDL particle number and composition. In Chapter 1, we described the difference between LDL cholesterol and apoB levels and outlined the mechanisms that link hypertriglyceridemia and the small, dense LDL and low HDL cholesterol. We will now consider how triglycerides, small, dense LDL and apoB are linked to risk.

The recently published AMORIS study was specifically designed to compare cholesterol and apoB as markers of the risk of death from myocardial infarction in 175 553 Swedes over a 6-year follow-up period. ApoB was superior to total or LDL cholesterol in every direct comparison. ApoB was predictive above and below the age of 70 years, whereas LDL cholesterol was predictive only below the age of 70. ApoB was predictive in men and women, whereas LDL cholesterol was predictive only in men. At all levels, apoB added information about risk, although this was particularly pronounced in individuals with LDL cholesterol below the median: < 3.73 mmol/L (150 mg/dL) in men and < 3.55 mmol/L (140 mg/dL) in women.

These are important results because they demonstrate that LDL particle number (that is, the level of apoB) is more powerful than total or LDL cholesterol level as an index of CHD risk. Just as important, when the findings of AMORIS are taken together with the findings of the Quebec Cardiovascular Study, they point to a better method to identify those at high risk than is commonly followed at the moment.

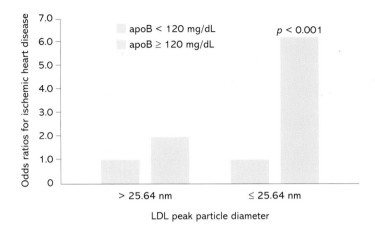

Figure 2.2 Interaction of apoB level and LDL particle size as determinants of CHD risk. Source: Lamarche et al. *Circulation* 1997;95:69.

Two of the most important results of the Quebec Cardiovascular Study are illustrated in Figure 2.2. This figure demonstrates that when apoB is increased, i.e. when LDL particle number is increased, but cholesterol-replete, normal-size LDL particles are present, risk is increased twofold. By contrast, when apoB is increased and small, dense LDL particles are present, risk is increased sixfold. Thus increased numbers of small, dense LDL particles are particularly dangerous. Because they are depleted in cholesterol, accurate diagnosis cannot be made by measurement of serum LDL cholesterol. Serum apoB measurement is necessary. Increased numbers of small, dense LDL particles are most likely to be present when triglycerides are raised and HDL is low.

These prospective data are consistent with data from several cross-sectional studies, and the following conclusions therefore seem reasonable.

- The three principal determinants of high risk are
  - high LDL particle number (apoB level)
  - small LDL particle size
  - low level of HDL.
- ApoB level is a measure of atherogenic particle number. At present, it is not practical to measure LDL particle size directly in clinical practice. Fortunately, LDL composition can be inferred from plasma

23

triglyceride level. HDL levels can be estimated by measuring either HDL cholesterol or apoAI.

- The total/HDL cholesterol or the apoB/apoAI ratios are the two simple summary indices of risk. Several studies indicate that apoB/apoAI is superior to total/HDL cholesterol, but unfortunately its measurement is not yet generally available to the clinician.

Pathogenesis of arteriosclerosis

LDL as the final common pathway. The frequency with which atherogenic lipoprotein particles encounter and enter the arterial wall is determined by their number and their size. LDL are more atherogenic than VLDL because the former are nine times more numerous and are smaller. On both these grounds, LDL qualify as the most dangerous of the atherogenic lipoproteins.

It is useful to think of LDL as the final common pathway to induce arteriosclerosis – that it is to say, most often, LDL plays a key role in the pathogenesis of the disease. This can occur in several ways. Some patients have marked hypercholesterolemia and thus a markedly increased LDL particle number, which alone may be sufficient over time to induce arterial disease. An example of this would be familial hypercholesterolemia (Chapter 3).

But the majority of patients destined to develop atherosclerosis do not fall into this group. Most have an only moderately elevated LDL particle number, or even a level that is normal for affluent Western societies. We have already mentioned the importance of LDL size, but there are often other factors which act to increase the atherogenic risk from LDL. Hypertension, diabetes and smoking are generally thought to be independent risk factors for disease, and that may be true statistically but not necessarily biologically. Biologically, these other risk factors modify the impact of the LDL on the arterial wall. For example, hypertension increases the likelihood that an LDL particle will be forced into the vessel wall. The vessel wall is also thickened, so that an LDL particle which gets embedded in it is less likely to get out and consequently is more likely to be harmful.

As we shall see, atherogenic dyslipoproteinemias are extremely common in type 2 diabetes; but in diabetes there are additional pathogenic factors at work. Glycation of the glycosaminoglycans of the vessel wall and the lipoprotein particles themselves increases the likelihood of an LDL particle sticking within the vessel wall and then being oxidized and promoting atherogenesis. The albuminuria common in diabetes may be one facet of a more generalized leakiness of blood vessels. The potential for oxidation is increased and antioxidant defenses frequently diminished in diabetes. Similarly, smoking provides a source of oxygen free radicals and of carbon monoxide which increases the permeability of the endothelial surface to LDL particles.

Age is actually the most powerful risk factor for vascular disease and fits nicely into this scheme as well. The risk of disease is proportional not only to the number of LDL particles in plasma and inversely to their size, but also to the duration of exposure. The longer a vessel wall is exposed, the more injurious events there will be.

We place this great emphasis on LDL because the evidence indicates LDL is the central risk factor for coronary disease. In so much of the world which does not consume the energetically excessive, fat-rich Western diet, despite high rates of smoking and hypertension the incidence of vascular disease is extremely low, because LDL levels are low. Nevertheless, even in these societies, a relationship to LDL can still be traced. The second reason is the mass of evidence now available from multiple clinical trials which unequivocally demonstrates that, at virtually all levels of LDL cholesterol, lowering LDL by pharmacological therapy significantly lowers coronary artery disease mortality and morbidity.

Atherogenesis: events in the arterial wall

Anitschov, the great Russian experimental pathologist, wrote in 1913 that 'there can be no atheroma without cholesterol'. Just as the epidemiological evidence points firmly in that direction, so does our recent understanding of the pathological processes that lead to coronary atherogenesis, and subsequent thrombosis and occlusion. Disturbingly, in parts of the world with high CHD rates, the earliest lesions, which give rise to later atheroma, are prevalent among children. These early lesions are the fatty streaks that are commonly present in the aortas of children unfortunate enough to succumb to some unrelated sudden death, such as an accident. Fatty streaks consist of collections of cells loaded with cytoplasmic droplets of cholesterol beneath the intimal surface of an artery (Figure 2.3). These cells are called foam cells and are usually macrophages that have internalized LDL from the tissue fluid in such quantities as to load their cytoplasm with cholesterol droplets. The initiating event in fatty streak formation is the passage of increased quantities of LDL across the endothelium of an artery into its wall. This is likely to occur at sites of turbulence, where there may be relative anoxia, when LDL levels are high and when the endothelium is damaged by, for example, hypertension, oxidation or glycation. Monocytes from the blood circulation are attracted to these sites by the damaged endothelium and themselves cross the endothelium to enter the subintimal space, where they take up LDL and assume the morphology of macrophages. Healthy, unmodified LDL is taken up only slowly, if at all, by macrophages. It must undergo some modification before it can excite foam cell formation. The modification that has attracted most recent interest has been oxidation.

Oxidation. Oxygen is two electrons short of having the same electron shell as inert neon. It forms stable compounds by sharing electrons from the outer shells of the atoms with which it reacts – for example, one from each of two hydrogen atoms to form water. Reactions of oxygen, including those catalyzed by enzymes, involve the production of an intermediate in which oxygen has acquired one additional electron in its outer shell, but has yet to receive the second to complete the reaction. At this stage, it is known as an oxygen free radical and is highly reactive, with its outer electron shell resembling that of fluorine. Oxygen free radicals are particularly reactive at the site of double carbon bonds in organic compounds. LDL has an abundance of these in the fatty acids of the phospholipids present in its outer envelope. Oxygen free-radical attack on these phospholipids leads to the formation of lipid peroxidation products. These react with, and damage, the apoB of LDL, altering its receptor-binding characteristics. This oxidatively modified LDL is rapidly taken up by macrophages through a class of receptors called scavenger receptors to form foam cells.

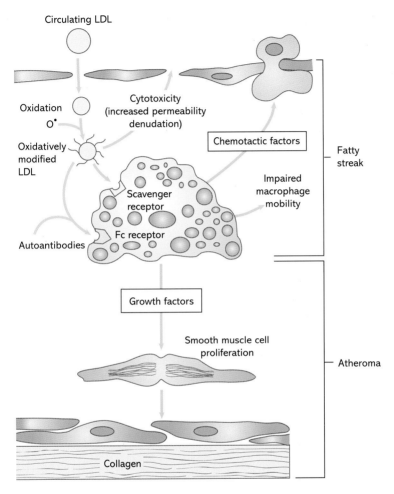

Figure 2.3 Atherogenesis: the fatty streak is characterized by lipid-laden macrophages (foam cells derived from blood monocytes attracted to the arterial subintima, where they engulf lipoproteins, such as oxidatively modified LDL). Conversion of the fatty streak to atheroma depends on the proliferation and differentiation of smooth-muscle cells into fibroblasts, the elaboration of collagen and repetition of the whole process. As the lesion progresses, necrosis of foam cells leaves behind extracellular lipid deposits; an overlying fibrous cap develops (see Figure 2.5). The actively growing point of the lesion where new foam cells are forming is in the shoulder at the junction between the atheromatous lesion and the normal arterial wall.

Oxygen free radicals:
- are present in cigarette smoke
- are formed during glycation reactions
- are generated deliberately by macrophages, for example to kill bacteria
- may leak from a variety of oxidative pathways.

Antioxidant mechanisms. LDL has its own fat-soluble antioxidants, which are dissolved in its central lipid droplet. They include:
- ubiquinone
- vitamin E (α- and β-tocopherol)
- β-carotene.

These are chain-breaking antioxidants; they themselves react more readily with oxygen free radicals than do phospholipids. Despite the widescale consumption of vitamin E and β-carotene in the belief that they will protect against atheroma, clinical trial evidence of such an effect is unconvincing. This is perhaps because when fat-soluble antioxidants are themselves oxidized, they offer no further protection against oxidation and may even behave as pro-oxidants.

HDL also appears to protect LDL against oxidative modification. It does so not by interfering with the formation of lipid peroxides on LDL, but by metabolizing them before they undergo spontaneous breakdown to form apoB-damaging substances. No means of enhancing this activity, which is largely due to the enzyme paraoxonase located on HDL, is yet known. The best policy for decreasing the production of oxidatively modified LDL is to reduce the quantity of LDL present in the circulation, or at least that of the subfractions of LDL which are most susceptible to oxidation.

Effects of oxidatively modified LDL. These are not confined to foam cell formation. Oxidatively modified LDL can also directly damage endothelial cells, stimulate the formation of autoantibodies, and excite macrophages and endothelial cells to secrete chemotactic factors that attract circulating monocytes. Foam cells themselves can produce growth factors that recruit smooth-muscle cells located further out in the aortic wall into the fatty streak region. These smooth-muscle cells differentiate into fibroblasts and lay down collagen. This response, which is clearly part of an inappropriately activated tissue repair process, leads to the development of the atheromatous plaque, the mature atheromatous lesion (Figure 2.4).

Plaque formation. The collagen elaborated by fibroblasts comes to overlie the macrophage foam cells, which undergo either necrosis or apoptosis. This results in the formation of a pool of extracellular cholesterol trapped beneath a fibrous cap. The shoulder of the atheromatous lesion (where the fibrous cap joins the normal arterial wall) continues to be active and it is here that active foam cell formation continues as the lesion advances across the inner surface of the artery (Figure 2.5). The fibrous cap is also at its most mechanically weak in this region; the secretion of collagenase from the macrophage

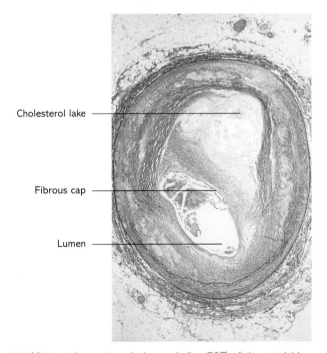

Figure 2.4 Mature atheromatous lesion occluding 70% of the arterial lumen. Reproduced courtesy of the Department of Pathological Sciences, Manchester Royal Infirmary, UK.

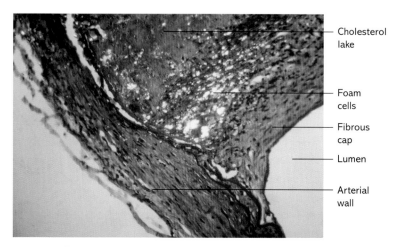

Cholesterol lake

Foam cells

Fibrous cap

Lumen

Arterial wall

Figure 2.5 The active shoulder region of a mature, cholesterol-rich plaque. At this site, the foam cells are clearly active (the orange-red material is lipid stained with Oil Red O, and pale intracellular cholesterol crystals are also present within the macrophages) and the fibrous cap is most vulnerable to rupture. Reproduced courtesy of the Department of Pathological Sciences, Manchester Royal Infirmary, UK.

foam cells may exacerbate this weakness. The part of the cap that ruptures is almost invariably in the shoulder of the plaque. Cholesterol-rich plaques are particularly liable to rupture their overlying fibrous cap. This becomes less likely as the quantity of fibrous tissue binding down the cap increases. Asymptomatic lesions, which occlude only 40–50% of the coronary artery lumen at a stage when they are particularly rich in cholesterol, may be more liable to rupture their caps than larger more fibrous lesions that obstruct the artery sufficiently to cause stable angina.

Rupture of a fibrous cap may lead to discharge of the cholesterol lake from beneath it. Should healing of the broken surface then occur uneventfully, a largely fibrous atheromatous lesion will result. However, if the victim of plaque rupture is unfortunate, thrombosis will occur at the raw site of the ruptured cap (Figure 2.6). Extension of this thrombosis will cause acute occlusion of the coronary artery lumen, resulting in myocardial infarction or unstable angina.

Factors that may ultimately determine the fate of a person harboring coronary atheroma include:

- those promoting plaque rupture, such as a high circulating concentration of LDL cholesterol (contributing to formation of plaques enriched in cholesterol relative to collagen and heightening foam cell activity in the vulnerable parts of the plaque) and/or sudden rises in blood pressure
- those that make thrombosis more likely, such as cigarette smoking and diabetes, which increase circulating plasma fibrinogen levels
- the extent of myocardial damage when occlusion occurs or the propensity of the ischemic myocardium to dysrhythmia.

The scale of the problem

The UK population probably has the highest serum cholesterol levels in the world. CHD rates in the west of Scotland and Northern Ireland have recently been exceeded by those of the Czech Republic, so it is

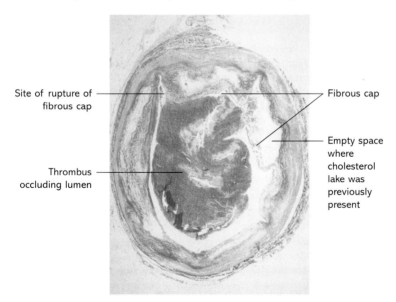

Figure 2.6 A ruptured plaque from which the cholesterol lake beneath the fibrous cap has discharged. A thrombus has formed at the raw endothelial surface of the rupture site, and the lumen is completely occluded. Reproduced courtesy of the Department of Pathological Sciences, Manchester Royal Infirmary, UK.

possible that other countries are in contention. Nevertheless, it is probably the worst single cause of ill health and premature death in the UK. Two thirds of the UK population have serum cholesterol levels exceeding the optimal upper limit for a population, 5.0 mmol/L (200 mg/dL). The situation is better in the USA, where both serum cholesterol and CHD rates are lower. They are not, however, sufficiently low that there can be any grounds for complacency.

A note on classification of hyperlipoproteinemias

The various forms of hyperlipoproteinemia used to be designated type I to type V depending on whether chylomicron triglyceride, VLDL triglyceride or both were elevated and whether LDL cholesterol was or was not raised as well. This convention has fallen into disuse. Now we distinguish

- combined hyperlipidemia if triglycerides and LDL cholesterol are elevated
- moderate or severe hypertriglyceridemia if triglycerides are raised but LDL cholesterol is normal
- high LDL cholesterol with normal triglycerides
- low HDL cholesterol with or without other abnormalities.

Epidemiology and pathophysiology – Key points

- The atherogenic lipoproteins, particularly LDL, form the final common pathway to the creation of atherosclerotic lesions.
- Blood pressure, diabetes mellitus, smoking and inflammation increase the entry of atherogenic lipoproteins into the arterial wall and increase the likelihood of plaque rupture.

Key references

Charlton J, Murphy M, Khaw K et al. Cardiovascular diseases. In: Charlton J et al., eds. *The Health of Adult Britain 1841–1994*, vol 2. London: The Stationery Office, 1997:60–81.

Charlton J, Quaife K. Trends in diet 1841–1994. In: Charlton J et al., eds. *The Health of Adult Britain 1841–1994*, vol 1. London: The Stationery Office, 1997:93–113.

Gordon DJ. Epidemiology of lipoproteins. In: Betteridge DJ et al., eds. *Lipoproteins in Health and Disease*. London: Arnold, 1999:587–95.

Law MR, Wald NJ, Thompson SG. By how much and how quickly does reduction in serum cholesterol concentration lower risk of ischaemic heart disease? *BMJ* 1994;308: 367–72.

Ross R. The pathogenesis of atherosclerosis: a perspective for the 1990s. *Nature* 1993;362:801–9.

Sniderman AD, Pedersen T, Kjekshus J. Putting low-density lipoproteins at center stage in atherogenesis. *Am J Cardiol* 1997;79:64–7.

Steinberg D. Low density lipoprotein oxidation and its pathobiological significance. *J Biol Chem* 1997; 272:20963–6.

Heterozygous familial hypercholesterolemia

Genetic basis. Familial hypercholesterolemia (FH) is the most common genetic disorder in Europe and the USA, affecting about 1 in 500 people in its heterozygous form. The existence of a dominantly inherited form of hypercholesterolemia causing tendon xanthomata has been recognized for 70 years. The nature of the genetic mutation causing the condition was not revealed, however, until 1974 when Goldstein and Brown in Dallas discovered the LDL receptor and found its expression to be diminished in fibroblasts from patients with FH. It is now known that the gene for the LDL receptor is located on chromosome 19.

The LDL receptor allows LDL to be taken up by cells from the tissue fluid. Newly synthesized receptors migrate to the cell surface where they can bind LDL. They move through the cell membrane to the region of the cell surface containing the coated pits, where invagination of the cell membrane is active. The invaginated membrane enters the cell cytoplasm as a vesicle containing a variety of receptors and their bound ligands. In the case of the LDL receptors, these are released back into the cytoplasm leaving any LDL they are carrying behind in the vesicle. They then travel back to the cell membrane so that the whole cycle may be repeated. This is believed to occur about every 10 minutes. The vesicles containing LDL fuse to form larger vesicles, called endosomes, into which enzymes are secreted that break down the apoB and esterified cholesterol to amino acids and free cholesterol, respectively; these can then diffuse out into the cytoplasm.

In FH, a mutation of the receptor prevents it from participating efficiently in LDL uptake, because it cannot be transported to the cell surface, cannot bind properly to LDL once it gets there, cannot be internalized, or is not released from the endosome. In FH heterozygotes, one of the LDL-receptor genes has a mutation; in homozygous FH, both do. Well before the discovery of the LDL-receptor defect, it was shown that the time LDL spent in the circulation before its removal was increased from the normal 2.5 days to about 4.5 days in heterozygotes and even longer in homozygotes (Figure 3.1). Impaired LDL uptake is the explanation for this observation.

A wide variety of mutations of the LDL receptor have been found to cause the clinical syndrome of FH in societies such as the UK and USA – more than 200 have been reported. In societies that have arisen relatively recently from a small number of early settlers or migrants, the frequency of FH may be more than 1 in 500, caused by a smaller number of different mutations. For example, 1 in 80 South Africans of Dutch or French descent have FH and the majority have one of only three different LDL-receptor mutations. Two of the mutations can be traced back to two of the early Dutch settlers and the other to a Huguenot migrant. A similar situation appears to exist among

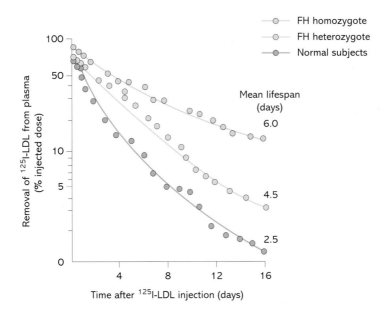

Figure 3.1 Radiolabeled LDL disappears from the circulation more slowly in patients with familial hypercholesterolemia than in normal controls. Data from Bilheimer et al. *J Clin Invest* 1979;64:524–33.

descendants of French Canadian settlers, and the high prevalence of FH in the Lebanon has sometimes been ascribed to an LDL-receptor mutation introduced by a Crusader. In families with members affected by FH, marriage to close relatives for cultural or religious reasons is also likely to increase greatly the likelihood of producing a family member with homozygous FH.

Diagnosis. FH can generally be diagnosed with ease if features of the clinical syndrome are carefully sought in people with hypercholesterolemia. Whether the FH genotype can be present in people without the clinical syndrome is debatable, as is the role of genetic testing. It seems highly likely, however, that people with the FH genotype and no clinical features of FH are rare, and it is by no means certain that they are at risk of premature CHD. Furthermore, because of the variety of mutations encountered in unrelated patients with FH, no simple, widely applicable means of genetic testing is feasible, except perhaps in a country such as South Africa where a much smaller number of different mutations exist.

It is important to emphasize that the introduction of lipid-lowering therapy is not the only reason for identifying heterozygotes for FH. The disorder is still not widely recognized. Therefore, when FH patients present with manifestations of CHD, they are often inappropriately managed if seen by physicians unfamiliar with the condition. There is a general disbelief that apparently fit, young people can have severe CHD. This usually leads to delay in investigations, particularly coronary angiography. Certainly exercise electrocardiography should be carried out promptly should symptoms that are in the least suggestive of CHD occur, and FH patients should be encouraged to report such symptoms. Coronary angiograms often reveal surprisingly extensive disease despite relatively minimal symptoms and should not be withheld. The pressure gradient across the aortic valve should be measured using echocardiography when a systolic murmur is present.

Cholesterol measurements. Serum cholesterol in heterozygous FH is raised from birth – normal mean serum cholesterol concentration in umbilical cord blood is only 1.7–2.0 mmol/L (68–80 mg/dL). However, screening using total serum cholesterol is not recommended at this stage because high HDL cholesterol (the dominant lipoprotein in fetal blood) is a much more common cause of high cord-blood cholesterol levels than FH. Serum cholesterol rises in the first year of life to a mean of 4.0 mmol/L (160 mg/dL; 95th percentile, 5.0 mmol/L or 200 mg/dL) and persists until the early teens with mean levels being similar in boys and girls before puberty. The normal range for serum cholesterol varies little with age during childhood; this allows a diagnostic threshold for childhood FH to be defined and explains why a total serum cholesterol above 6.5 mmol/L (260 mg/dL) identifies 95% of heterozygotes and only 2.5% of unaffected children. It is, of course, important to confine cholesterol measurements to the children of affected parents, so that the chances of the condition occurring are 1 in 2. If children in general were screened, the chance of finding a heterozygote would be 1 in 500, so even a 2.5% false-positive rate would falsely identify ten unaffected children for every one affected. In almost all affected children, the serum cholesterol exceeds 7.0 mmol/L (280 mg/dL). In families with FH, measuring cholesterol in childhood can lead to uncertainty if serum cholesterol is 5.5–7.0 mmol/L (220–280 mg/dL), particularly if the family is already on a cholesterol-lowering diet. The diagnosis cannot then be made or excluded with complete confidence, and repeated measurements over time are required.

With advancing age, the serum cholesterol in FH, as in the general population, increases. In heterozygous FH, it is generally double what it would have been in the absence of the LDL-receptor mutation. For example, in a young adult woman whose serum cholesterol might have been only 4.0 mmol/L (160 mg/dL) had she not inherited the disorder, a level of 8.0 mmol/L (320 mg/dL) may indicate FH. By adulthood, the serum cholesterol in heterozygous FH is, however, typically in the range 9.0–14.0 mmol/L (360–560 mg/dL).

Tendon xanthomata, corneal arcus and xanthelasmata. Tendon xanthomata are the diagnostic hallmarks of FH. The only other causes of these, cerebrotendinous xanthomata and phytosterolemia, are so rare that for practical purposes, in the presence of tendon xanthomata, the diagnosis of FH is never really in doubt. Xanthomata are localized infiltrates of lipid-containing foam cells that histologically resemble atheroma.

Corneal arcus (Figure 3.2) and xanthelasmata (Figure 3.3) are not specific for FH, though they often occur much earlier in life in people with FH than in those with the more common polygenic type of hypercholesterolemia (see Chapter 4). Corneal arcus, for example, in the late teens or twenties may well indicate FH. On the other hand, xanthelasmata not infrequently occur in women during their first pregnancy when, at other times, their serum cholesterol is not particularly high. A great many FH heterozygotes with obvious tendon xanthomata do not have corneal arcus until much later, however, and will never develop xanthelasmata. Tendon xanthomata should, therefore, be sought in all patients with hypercholesterolemia, regardless of the presence of corneal arcus or xanthelasmata.

The most common sites for tendon xanthomata are in the tendons overlying the knuckles and in the Achilles tendons (Figure 3.4). Less commonly, they may be found in the extensor hallucis longus and triceps tendons, and occasionally others. It is quite common to find xanthomata on the tibial tuberosity at the site of insertion of the patellar tendon (Figure 3.5). These are called subperiosteal xanthomata and are firmly attached to the bone.

It must be emphasized that the skin overlying tendon xanthomata and subperiosteal xanthomata has a normal color and does not appear yellow. The cholesterol accumulation is deep within the tendons, and much of the swelling is fibrous. The xanthomata feel hard. Those in the Achilles tendons show a tendency to become inflamed, and many patients with FH will, if asked, give a history of earlier episodes of Achilles tenosynovitis. Xanthomata in the tendons on the dorsum of the hands are generally nodular or fusiform and, because they often overlie the knuckles (particularly when the fist is clenched) and are as hard as bone, physicians may miss them. The hand should be examined with the fingers extended – the xanthomata move back and can be moved from side to side. Achilles tendon xanthomata may be obvious, if sought, because of thickening, swelling, irregularity or nodularity of the tendon on visual inspection. They may, however, be more subtle, with the nodularity on the tendon becoming obvious only on palpation.

Family history. The other striking feature of FH is often the adverse family history of CHD, though in societies such as those of northern

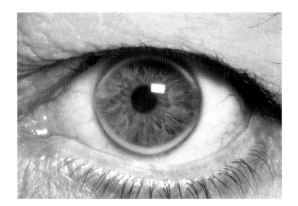

Figure 3.2
Corneal arcus.

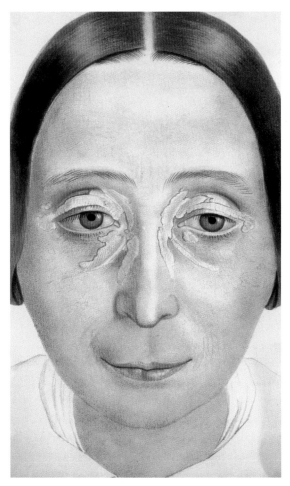

Figure 3.3 Eliza Parachute, the first patient described with xanthelasmata (*Addison & Gull Guy's Hospital Reports* 1851;series II, 7:265–70).

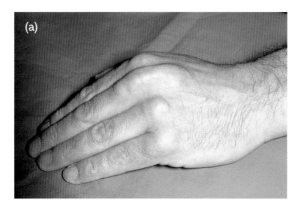

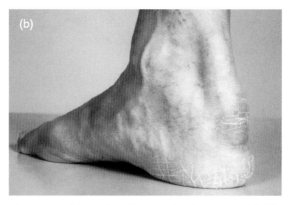

Figure 3.4 Tendon xanthomata on (a) the knuckle, reproduced courtesy of Dr JH Barth, Leeds General Infirmary, UK, and (b) the Achilles tendon.

Europe and North America, a family history of early-onset CHD is of course common in the general population. Nonetheless, because FH is treatable, its diagnosis should always be sought when such a history is encountered. It is hypercholesterolemia that is inherited in FH, not necessarily the propensity to premature CHD. In some families, FH seems particularly devastating, causing CHD in men in their twenties and women before the menopause. In others, men are unaffected until late middle age and occasionally older, and women may survive to extreme old age with minimal CHD symptoms.

The general level of CHD risk can be appreciated from Table 3.1. The median age for the development of CHD in men is around 50 years. Typically, affected women in the same family develop CHD

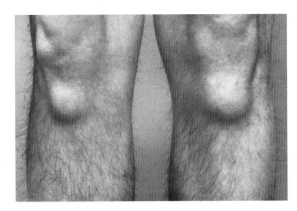

Figure 3.5
Subperiosteal
xanthomata over
tibial tuberosities.

about 9 years later than their male relatives with FH. Furthermore, the penetrance of FH judged in terms of CHD risk tends to breed true in families. Thus it is striking how often one encounters a family in whom all the affected male members developed CHD at a similar age and their affected female relatives some 9 years later. This can be helpful clinically – for example, in making decisions as to the age at which to introduce lipid-lowering medication. If the family history is particularly adverse, this might be as early as adolescence in male heterozygotes. In other families in which the hypercholesterolemia is pursuing a more benign course, medication may be started later; for example, in many women from such families, the introduction of cholesterol-lowering medication can safely be left until they are in their thirties or later.

Tenosynovitis. In addition to Achilles tendonitis, a more generalized tenosynovitis may occur in FH. This is most commonly seen when cholesterol is lowered abruptly by, for example, partial ileal bypass, but it can also occur when cholesterol is lowered with other therapies, such as statins, when it may be wrongly attributed to the drug itself. It is due to the mobilization of cholesterol widely deposited in the tendons and periarticular tissues, and is akin to the exacerbations of gout that may accompany the mobilization of uric acid when allopurinol is introduced for the first time.

Homozygous familial hypercholesterolemia
This is rare when it occurs by chance. The odds of two unrelated heterozygotes marrying is 1 in 250 000 (unless, of course, they meet at

TABLE 3.1

CHD incidence and mortality associated with untreated heterozygous FH*

Age (years)	CHD incidence (%)		CHD mortality (%)	
	Men	Women	Men	Women
< 30	5	0	0	0
30–39	22	2	7	0
40–49	48	7	25	1
50–59	80	51	52	15
60–69	100	75	78	23

*Compilation of studies in the UK (Slack. *Lancet* 1969;2:1380–2), the USA (Stone et al. *Circulation* 1974;49:476–88) and France (Beaumont et al. *Atherosclerosis* 1976;24:441–50)

a lipid clinic) and the chances of them having a child who is homozygous is 1 in 4, making the theoretical incidence of homozygous FH 1 in a million. The chances of a marriage between heterozygotes is greatly increased when there is, for example, a tradition of first-cousin marriage. In such circumstances, both of the LDL-receptor mutations in homozygotes are likely to be the same, and the affected person is a true homozygote. Homozygotes arising from random union are likely to have a different LDL-receptor mutation on each chromosome and are, in reality, compound heterozygotes (though they are classified as homozygotes).

Signs. Homozygous FH is always a serious problem. Serum cholesterol levels are almost invariably greater than 15 mmol/L (600 mg/dL) and can be as high as 30 mmol/L (1200 mg/dL). Xanthomata develop in childhood. In addition to florid tendon xanthomata of the type already described, orange-yellow cutaneous planar xanthomata develop, particularly in the popliteal and antecubital fossae, buttocks and in the webs between the fingers (Figure 3.6). They may develop on the palms of the hands and the fronts of the knees during crawling. Polyarthralgia is common and supravalvar aortic stenosis can cause sudden death.

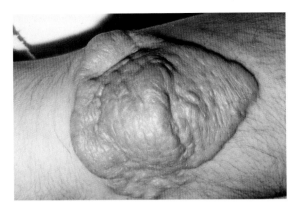

Figure 3.6 Subcutaneous planar xanthoma in the antecubital fossa. Reproduced courtesy of Dr JP Miller, University Hospital of South Manchester, UK.

Most homozygotes develop angina of effort in childhood due to the aortic stenosis and coronary atheroma. Myocardial infarction has been recorded as early as at 2 years, and life expectancy does not usually extend beyond the early twenties. The very worst prognosis seems to occur when both LDL-receptor mutations are of the type that completely prevents LDL receptors appearing on the cell surface.

Management

Heterozygous FH. The statin drugs represent a major advance in the management of FH. Most people with heterozygous FH can now achieve serum cholesterol levels below 7.0 mmol/L (280 mg/dL) and some even below 5.0 mmol/L (200 mg/dL). The most potent of the statins may be required at maximum dose in patients with the higher cholesterol levels. Occasionally the therapeutic response is still inadequate, in which case a bile-acid sequestrating agent is the most logical addition. Nicotinic acid in doses up to 7 g daily is also effective, but must be carefully monitored and is rarely acceptable to patients because of the severe flushing it invariably produces. Partial ileal bypass is often successful in decreasing serum cholesterol, but has been used less often since the advent of statins.

Homozygous FH. The cholesterol-lowering effect achieved with medication in homozygous FH is generally disappointing, with the

43

exception of that achieved with atorvastatin, which can decrease serum cholesterol by up to 30%. Even then, substantial hypercholesterolemia remains. Plasmapheresis or LDL apheresis is the best approach to correcting this. Generally the procedure must be carried out every 2 weeks. Liver transplantation has also met with some success. This introduces normal donor hepatic LDL receptors. The LDL-receptor gene can be expressed in transfected LDL-receptor knockout mice, lowering serum cholesterol, albeit only briefly before it is cleared from the cell nuclei along with viral DNA. Homozygous FH will be one of the first genetic disorders to be treated by this technique as soon as a vector that allows foreign DNA to persist in mammalian cells becomes available.

Genetic counseling

There is no need to suggest that a patient with heterozygous FH should limit their family as long as their partner is not also a heterozygote. It is advisable to check the partner's serum cholesterol to establish this. Although one child in two of a heterozygote for FH with a non-FH partner will themselves be FH heterozygotes, the prospect for improved treatment is great and the condition not generally so severe as to suggest that such individuals will not benefit from their life. However, depending on the family history, it may be sensible that FH patients do not wait until the bloom of youth is too far behind them before starting their families, because of the devastating effect the death of a parent can have on young children.

Familial defective apoB

The FH phenotype is usually caused by an LDL-receptor mutation. Rarely, however, the same FH syndrome is caused because apoB has a mutation that interferes with binding, thus producing a similar defect in LDL catabolism. This is called familial defective apoB (FDB). It is most commonly due to an amino-acid substitution at position 3500. This mutation has a frequency of about 1 in 600 in the general population, though it does not generally produce a particularly severe hyperlipidemia. It has, however, been estimated that perhaps as many as 4% of people with clinical FH have FDB. Their hypercholesterolemia appears to respond more easily to treatment than is generally the case in FH.

Autosomal-recessive hypercholesterolemia

A condition called autosomal-recessive hypercholesterolemia, so far described only in people of Sardinian extraction, produces a clinical phenotype intermediate between homozygous and heterozygous FH. It involves a defect in LDL catabolism not mediated through mutation of the LDL receptor genes, but through a gene involved in the internalization of LDL from the cell surface by endocytosis once it has bound to its receptor.

Other mutations leading to FH

Currently, about half of the patients in the UK and USA with a clinical diagnosis of heterozygous FH have identifiable mutations of the LDL receptor; a much smaller proportion have FDB. It is possible that genetic techniques are failing to detect LDL-receptor mutations in some FH patients. It is also possible that another gene or genes involved in LDL catabolism will be found that, when they undergo mutation, explain the presence of FH in some patients. Although this adds considerable interest to the subject, we already have sufficient knowledge of the natural history of the clinical syndrome of FH to treat it with vigor.

CHD susceptibility

CHD is far and away the most common manifestation of atheroma in heterozygous FH. Atheromatous deposits may also occur in the root of the aorta and can extend into the aortic valve cusps; these occur particularly in homozygous FH, but also in as many as 30% of heterozygotes. This form of supravalvar aortic stenosis and aortic sclerosis may be the cause of an aortic systolic murmur. Some patients also develop carotid and intracerebral atheroma, though not as frequently as CHD. Femoropopliteal atheroma is also less common than CHD and is really only encountered in cigarette smokers with FH.

There has been much speculation as to why some families with FH are more susceptible to CHD than others. The nature of the mutation might itself be important, because some mutations will more severely compromise LDL uptake than others. The particular combination of mutations certainly influences the severity of homozygous FH, but this is less clear in heterozygous FH. Indeed, neither the pre-treatment LDL cholesterol level nor the extent and size of tendon xanthomata is clearly related to prognosis in FH. Serum HDL cholesterol is, however, related to the likelihood of CHD in FH. Serum HDL cholesterol is generally lower than expected in FH; prognosis is often bad in families where this is most obvious. Usually in FH, only the serum cholesterol is raised as a consequence of the increase in LDL. Triglycerides are elevated in a minority of patients, though seldom to more than 4.0 mmol/L (360 mg/dL). This too has been associated with a worse prognosis. These people are often obese, and obesity can increase serum cholesterol, sometimes even to 20 mmol/L (800 mg/dL) or more.

Obesity is generally uncommon in FH – in contrast to all other hyperlipidemias, in which obesity is over-represented. Hypertension and diabetes mellitus are noticeably uncommon in FH; again, this is unlike other hyperlipoproteinemias. Cigarette smoking may be more common in some families with a worse prognosis, and socio-economic deprivation almost certainly worsens the outlook. Co-inheritance of the apoE4 allele or alleles or of high serum Lp(a) may also be associated with a worse prognosis.

Familial (monogenic) hypercholesterolemia – Key points

- Heterozygous FH carries a particularly high risk of CHD and requires early treatment.
- Diagnosis therefore is critical. Fortunately, FH families have a distinctive clinical picture.
- Homozygous FH fortunately is much rarer but unfortunately remains a treatment challenge.

Key references

Arca M, Zuliani G, Wilund K et al. Autosomal recessive hypercholesterolaemia in Sardinia, Italy, and mutations in ARH: a clinical and molecular genetic analysis. *Lancet* 2002;359: 841–7.

Durrington PN. Familial hypercholesterolaemia. In: *Hyperlipidaemia, Diagnosis and Management.* Oxford: Butterworth-Heinemann, 1995:108–39.

Goldstein JL, Hobbs HH, Brown MS. Familial hypercholesterolaemia. In: Scriver CR et al., eds. *The Metabolic and Molecular Bases of Inherited Disease,* 7th edn, vol 2. New York: McGraw Hill, 1995:1981–2030.

Polygenic hypercholesterolemia and combined hypercholesterolemia and hypertriglyceridemia (combined hyperlipidemia) are much more common causes of an elevated LDL cholesterol than FH. In Europe and North America, FH probably accounts for no more than 3% of men dying of CHD before the age of 60. We will present both polygenic hypercholesterolemia and combined hyperlipidemia from the conventional point of view, but also take the opportunity to demonstrate what can be added by knowledge of apoB level and hence particle number.

Polygenic hypercholesterolemia

Figure 4.1a illustrates schematically a normal complement of VLDL and LDL particles. There are nine times more LDL than VLDL particles, and most of the LDL particles are cholesterol replete. Because particle number is normal, total cholesterol, triglyceride, LDL cholesterol and apoB are all normal.

Figure 4.1b illustrates the lipoprotein profile in a patient with polygenic hypercholesterolemia. The patient either has a normal number of VLDL particles or, if they are increased as a consequence of overproduction, they contain less triglyceride. Plasma triglyceride levels are not therefore increased. However, there is an increased number of LDL particles, which are normal in composition. Therefore, total cholesterol, LDL cholesterol and apoB are all increased.

In most instances, the increased LDL is due to overproduction of LDL particles rather than impaired clearance. It is interesting that VLDL secretion can be increased in the absence of hypertriglyceridemia. These individuals may be particularly adept at hydrolyzing triglycerides in the periphery or they may secrete a relatively triglyceride-poor VLDL. In either case, the conversion of VLDL to LDL would remain relatively efficient. Overproduction of LDL would lead to increased LDL particle number because the capacity of even the normal LDL pathway to remove LDL particles from plasma is limited. The level of small, dense LDL is generally not increased in these patients. The risk of coronary disease is increased but not as markedly as in combined hyperlipidemia.

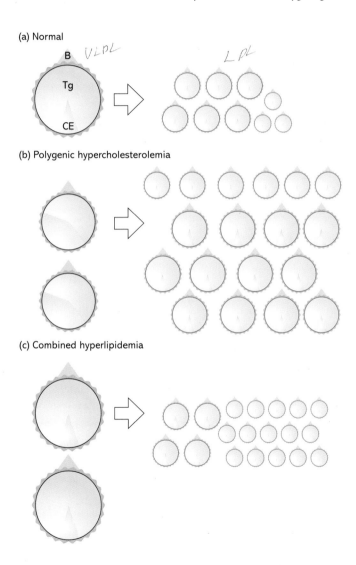

Figure 4.1 Lipoprotein profiles: (a) normal; (b) polygenic hypercholesterolemia; (c) combined hyperlipidemia. Tg, triglyceride; CE, cholesteryl ester; B, apolipoprotein B.

Combined hyperlipidemia

This is the commonest dyslipoproteinemia in patients with premature vascular disease. It is also among the most common dyslipoproteinemias in patients with type 2 diabetes and/or abdominal obesity. Furthermore, it is the characteristic dyslipoproteinemia of familial combined hyperlipidemia, the commonest familial dyslipoproteinemia associated with premature coronary artery disease.

Figure 4.1c illustrates the typical lipoprotein profile in these patients. Both VLDL and LDL particle numbers are increased, as is that of small, dense LDL. This produces hypertriglyceridemia and increased LDL cholesterol. Because most LDL particles are cholesterol-depleted, the apoB and therefore the LDL particle number is even higher than would be predicted from the LDL cholesterol. Note that HDL cholesterol also is often low in these patients, further increasing risk.

The pathophysiology of combined hyperlipidemia runs as follows. Compared with normal adipose tissue, the adipose tissue of these patients takes up and stores a smaller proportion of the dietary fatty acids that are released from chylomicrons by LPL. Thus, during the postprandial period, there is increased delivery of exogenous fatty acids to the liver. During fasting, there tends to be excessive release of fatty acids from adipose tissue, which of course also leads to increased delivery of fatty acids to the liver. Increased delivery of fatty acids results in increased hepatic triglyceride and cholesterol synthesis and therefore increased secretion rate of VLDL particles.

Reduced fatty acid trapping by adipose tissue is much more common in abdominal or male pattern obesity than in peripheral or female pattern obesity. Reduced fatty acid trapping and obesity would appear to be incompatible, but the contradiction is illusory. Fatty acid trapping describes the rate at which fatty acids enter adipose tissue. If fatty acid trapping is reduced, fewer fatty acids enter initially from chylomicrons, and this results in the synthesis and secretion of extra VLDL particles. Therefore, there is a second chance for fatty acids to enter the adipose tissue. Adipose is the only tissue with a substantial capacity to store fatty acids. Therefore, whenever fatty acids are ingested or produced in excess of metabolic need, adipose tissue mass will necessarily expand.

Decreased fatty acid trapping by adipose tissue produces other clinically important abnormalities. Elevated triglycerides and elevated apoB have been shown to be precursors of type 2 diabetes. Why should that be? The answer is likely to lie in the multiple adverse effects of fatty acids on glucose and insulin metabolism. Excess fatty acids cause insulin resistance: first because they oppose insulin-induced glucose uptake by muscle, and second because they inhibit the normal insulin-mediated suppression of hepatic VLDL secretion. This puts greater demand on the pancreas to maintain higher insulin levels to overcome these effects – a demand which individuals susceptible to diabetes cannot meet.

Familial combined hyperlipidemia (FCHL)

Originally, FCHL was thought to be a dominantly inherited hyperlipidemia closely associated with CHD, but differing from FH in that both hypercholesterolemia and hypertriglyceridemia were running within the same family and occurring singly or in combination in individual members. That is, within an affected family, there were, with roughly equal frequency, those with a combined increase in cholesterol and triglycerides, those with an increase in triglycerides only, and those with an increase in cholesterol only. In the original series of studies, this disorder was at least ten times more common than FH.

Subsequent research has not supported the concept of simple dominant inheritance, although genetic factors are clearly at work in affected families. FCHL remains an important clinical syndrome even though it is less easy to define than FH. In contrast to FH, hyperlipidemia does not generally appear in subjects with FCHL until early middle age, although an elevated apoB may be present much earlier. In addition, hypertension and hyperinsulinemia and/or hyperglycemia are commonly associated with FCHL, but not with FH. FCHL, like polygenic hypercholesterolemia, but again unlike FH, has as its root cause overproduction of VLDL, even in those affected individuals whose serum triglycerides are not raised.

Diagnosis of FCHL. Affected subjects may be normolipidemic, hypertriglyceridemic, hypercholesterolemic, or hypertriglyceridemic and

51

hypercholesterolemic, but all have an elevated apoB and small, dense LDL.

The elevated apoB is the consequence of increased secretion of VLDL particles. Depending on the composition of the VLDL secreted by the liver, and probably more importantly on the peripheral activity of LPL, plasma triglycerides may be normal or elevated. They are usually, however, greater than 1.5 mmol/L (130 mg/dL). Whether total and LDL cholesterol are normal or elevated depends on (a) the number of small, dense LDL that are present, (b) just how cholesterol-depleted they are and (c) the efficiency of the LDL pathway. It must be emphasized that the prime target of therapy in these patients is to reduce the atherogenic particle number – that is, to reduce the elevated plasma apoB.

Pathogenesis of FCHL. Much remains to be learned about the pathogenesis of FCHL. We think it is unlikely that a single gene will be responsible. Rather, any of several genes, individually or collectively, that impinge on a critical metabolic process are likely to be the culprits. Attention has focused on the effectiveness of fatty acid trapping by adipose tissue (see, for example, page 50). The two key players in this process are insulin and ASP. A major objective for research must be to understand the mechanisms which regulate the responsiveness of adipocytes to these two key peptides. Reduced uptake and storage of fatty acids in the postprandial period will produce increased delivery of fatty acids to the liver. This, in turn, will lead to increased secretion of VLDL particles by the liver and then to increased numbers of small, dense LDL.

Role of diet

Obesity and a high-fat diet (particularly one high in saturated fat) are probably the major reasons for the enormous variations worldwide in the prevalence of polygenic hypercholesterolemia and combined hyperlipidemia. Undoubtedly, however, individual responses to diet vary tremendously, and there is probably a complex interplay between dietetic and genetic factors in the genesis of the disorders.

There is an impression that dietary modification aimed at lowering cholesterol in middle age in societies in which serum cholesterol is high does not reduce it to the extent that might be expected. Whether this is simply a matter of non-compliance with diet or represents some permanent change in metabolism caused by a high-fat diet in early life is at present uncertain.

Physical signs in polygenic hypercholesterolemia and combined hyperlipidemia

Tendon xanthomata are absent in both disorders. Their presence in a patient with combined hyperlipidemia highly favors a diagnosis of the unusual co-occurrence of FH and hypertriglyceridemia. Obesity, particularly android obesity, is common in patients with combined hyperlipidemia. Xanthelesmata or corneal arcus occurs in all types of hypercholesterolemia. In patients with both hypercholesterolemia and hypertriglyceridemia, tuberoeruptive or striate palmar xanthomata generally indicate that the patient has type III hyperlipoproteinemia (see Chapter 6). Eruptive xanthomata are associated with severe hypertriglyceridemia with hyperchylomicronemia.

Polygenic hypercholesterolemia and combined hyperlipidemia – Key points

- Polygenic hypercholesterolemia and combined hyperlipidemia are two of the commonest, and therefore two of the most important, atherogenic dyslipoproteinemias.
- All other things being equal, the prognosis of combined hyperlipidemia is worse than that of polygenic hypercholesterolemia.
- Individuals with either phenotype may come from a family with familial combined hyperlipidemia.

Key references

Durrington P. Lipid and lipoprotein disorders. In: Weatherall DJ et al., eds. *Oxford Textbook of Medicine*, 3rd edn, vol 2. Oxford: Oxford University Press, 1996:1399–415.

Jarvik GP, Austin MA, Brunzell JD. Familial combined hyperlipidaemia. In: Betteridge DJ et al., eds. *Lipoproteins in Health and Disease*. London: Arnold, 1999:693–9.

Sniderman AD, Zhang XJ, Cianflone K. Governance of the concentration of plasma LDL: a reevaluation of the LDL receptor paradigm. *Atherosclerosis* 2000;148:215–29.

Treatment is necessary to avoid the risk of acute pancreatitis in extreme hypertriglyceridemia. The association of hypertriglyceridemia with CHD is complex, however, and CHD risk is not necessarily dependent on the triglyceride level. This chapter examines separately patients with moderate hypertriglyceridemia, 2.3–10 mmol/L (200–900 mg/dL), and those with higher levels. There is no sharp division between these groups, however. Some people with apparently moderate fasting hypertriglyceridemia have the capacity, under certain circumstances, to develop gross hypertriglyceridemia leading to acute pancreatitis; others who habitually have serum triglyceride values of more than 30 mmol/L (2700 mg/dL) can live to a ripe old age without complications.

Moderate hypertriglyceridemia

The upper limit of normal values for fasting serum triglycerides is generally quoted as 2.3 mmol/L (200 mg/dL), although the 95th percentiles for the UK and the US populations are closer to 3 mmol/L (270 mg/dL). On the other hand, an argument can be made for a value of 1.5 mmol/L (130 mg/dL) as being the cut-off point since above this level small, dense LDL particles become common whereas below it they are not.

In univariate analyses of epidemiological studies, serum triglycerides are often stronger predictors of CHD risk than serum cholesterol. There is, however, a strong inverse relationship between serum triglyceride and HDL cholesterol concentrations. This largely explains why inclusion of HDL cholesterol in risk prediction substantially eliminates the effects of triglycerides on risk. Nevertheless, some meta-analyses have shown that triglycerides still confer significant independent risk even after taking HDL cholesterol into account.

Statistical analyses have their limitations. They cannot infallibly identify cause and effect. In this case, the usual explanation for the low HDL cholesterol is core lipid exchange with the triglyceride-rich lipoprotein (see Chapter 2). If hypertriglyceridemia produces low HDL cholesterol, it makes no clinical sense therefore to conclude that HDL cholesterol is important and triglycerides are not.

Forms of moderate pure hypertriglyceridemia. By definition, all these patients have a normal LDL cholesterol level, but that is not to say that all patients with moderate hypertriglyceridemia are the same. There are two forms: one with a normal apoB and one with an elevated apoB. The distinction is important because a series of studies have shown that risk is markedly increased in the latter and only moderately increased, if at all, in the former. Unfortunately, the two forms cannot be accurately distinguished by measurement of lipid values. Also, as will be reviewed in the therapy section, the adequacy of statin therapy is best judged by the level of apoB, not by the concentration of LDL cholesterol.

ATPIII, the latest consensus report from the USA, has recommended that non-HDL cholesterol (total cholesterol minus HDL cholesterol) be calculated in these patients and used rather than LDL cholesterol as the main index of risk and the target for statin therapy. And indeed, there is a reasonable overall correlation between non-HDL cholesterol and apoB. However, there is far from perfect agreement: there is only a moderate difference in non-HDL cholesterol between the two groups, but there is a major difference in apoB.

The difference in risk between the two forms of hypertriglyceridemia can be understood from Figure 5.1 Hypertriglyceridemia with a normal apoB (Figure 5.1a) is characterized by larger, triglyceride-enriched VLDL particles. VLDL particle number is not increased and therefore LDL particle number is not increased. By contrast, hypertriglyceridemia with an elevated apoB (Figure 5.1b) is characterized by increased numbers of VLDL particles with normal composition. The increased VLDL particle number produces hypertriglyceridemia and increased numbers of small, dense LDL particles. It is this second form – hypertriglyceridemia with an elevated apoB – that is one of the most common manifestations of familial combined hyperlipidemia (see Chapter 4).

Drug treatment. There is no evidence that therapy aimed at reducing triglycerides in patients whose cholesterol is below 5 mmol/L

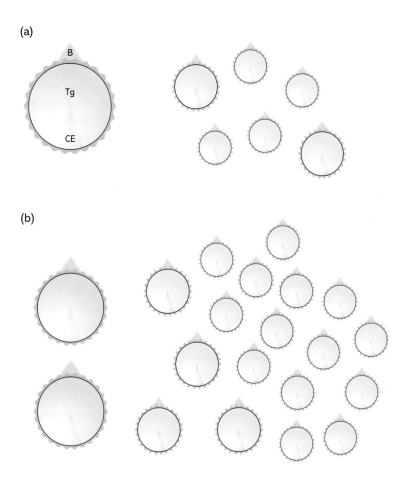

Figure 5.1 Lipoprotein profiles for two forms of hypertriglyceridemia: (a) with normal apoB; (b) the higher-risk form with elevated apoB. This latter form, characterized by elevated levels of VLDL and small, dense LDL, is one of the most common manifestations of familial combined hyperlipidemia. Tg, triglyceride; CE, cholesteryl ester; B, apolipoprotein B.

(200 mg/dL) is of benefit in patients without symptomatic coronary disease. As will be reviewed, it may be of benefit in patients with coronary disease although no significant reduction in mortality has been demonstrated. In patients without overt coronary disease, the overall risk should be calculated as will be set out in Chapter 10.

Before making the decision to introduce lipid-lowering drugs in hypertriglyceridemia, secondary causes should be sought and dietary advice given. In particular, excess alcohol consumption, liver disease and diabetes mellitus should be excluded.

Statins. When serum triglycerides are only moderately elevated, up to say 5.0 mmol/L (450 mg/dL), a statin may be the best first-line treatment. In addition to their cholesterol-lowering effect, statins also decrease triglycerides, and there is strong evidence that they prevent CHD, generally without adverse effects (which is not known with the same degree of certainty for some other lipid-lowering drugs).

For patients whose hypertriglyceridemia is too severe to respond to statin drugs, fish oil (or more concentrated omega–3 fatty acid preparations), fibrates and nicotinic acid should be considered.

Fish oil (omega–3 fatty acids) combined with a statin often decreases triglyceride levels satisfactorily. Fish oil has no cholesterol-decreasing effect. Although there is evidence that fish oil decreases CHD risk, this is not as strong as in the case of statins. It should not, therefore, be used alone.

Fibrates can be used as sole therapies, though their cholesterol-lowering effect is seldom adequate to achieve therapeutic targets for LDL cholesterol levels in, for example, myocardial infarction survivors. Indeed, in some patients with relatively low LDL cholesterol levels, these may initially increase on fibrate therapy.

Nicotinic acid is particularly effective at lowering both triglyceride and cholesterol levels. However, daily doses of several grams are generally required and at this level nicotinic acid has many side-effects (see Chapter 9).

Diet. Obesity is common in all types of hypertriglyceridemia, in which case dietary advice should be directed at weight reduction. In those who are not overweight, or who fail to lose weight, generally restricting saturated fats is more effective than advice to restrict carbohydrate intake. Restriction of refined carbohydrate is, however, sensible.

For patients to lose weight, decreases in overall fat intake may be required. In the case of severe hypertriglyceridemia, when the contribution of chylomicrons is significant, a restriction in all types of fat intake is essential. Under these circumstances, carbohydrate intake may have to be increased in lean patients. Many patients with hypertriglyceridemia are overtly diabetic. Others are glucose intolerant or will become so over the next few years. Weight reduction and dietary fat restriction improve glucose tolerance more effectively than carbohydrate restriction, because both measures decrease insulin resistance. It is insulin resistance that is generally the cause of diabetes or glucose intolerance in hypertriglyceridemia, particularly when associated with CHD.

Effect of β-blockers. The indications for β-blockers should be reviewed, particularly if the hypertriglyceridemia is marked. If β-blockers are clearly indicated, as in patients with established CHD, bear in mind that we do not yet know whether minor elevations of triglycerides produced by β-blockers are harmful and thus whether any form of treatment is required. Marked elevation of triglycerides should be treated, however, in patients who cannot discontinue β-blockers.

Severe hypertriglyceridemia (types I and V)

Diagnosis and underlying mechanism. In any circumstance where serum triglycerides exceed 10 mmol/L (900 mg/dL), chylomicrons will be major contributors to the hyperlipidemia, even when the patient is fasting. Chylomicrons and VLDL compete for the same clearance mechanism in the circulation (lipoprotein lipase). The lipoprotein phenotype is usually type V. This severe hypertriglyceridemia generally occurs when an increase in hepatic VLDL production, either familial or secondary to, for example, obesity, diabetes, alcohol abuse or estrogen administration, is associated with decreased triglyceride clearance. This again may be genetic or acquired: for example, in hypothyroidism, β-blockade or diabetes mellitus (diabetes can cause both overproduction of VLDL and decreased LPL activity).

With the clearance mechanism already overloaded with VLDL, the rise in serum triglyceride levels when chylomicrons enter the circulation following a fatty meal may be dramatic, and the chylomicrons may spend days rather than hours in the circulation. The serum takes on the appearance of milk (Figure 5.2), and triglyceride levels may exceed

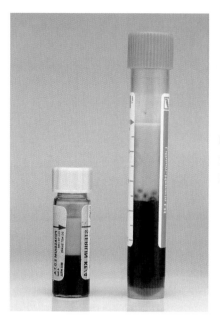

Figure 5.2 Milky serum from a patient with severe (type V) hyperlipoproteinemia.

100 mmol/L (9000 mg/dL). A patient who might otherwise have a fasting serum triglyceride level of 5 mmol/L (450 mg/dL) can, with the injudicious use of alcohol or the development of diabetes, achieve extraordinarily high serum triglyceride levels. Overall, the frequency of severe hypertriglyceridemia is probably no more than 1 in 1000 in adults, and lower in children.

Familial lipoprotein lipase (LPL) deficiency. Rarely, severe hypertriglyceridemia is caused by familial LPL deficiency, a genetic deficiency in LPL activity. This is inherited as an autosomal-recessive trait. It is usually due to mutation in the lipoprotein lipase gene, leading to defective function or production of the enzyme, but occasionally it results from a genetic deficiency of apoCII, the activator of LPL.

Severe hypertriglyceridemia may present during childhood. Occasionally in children and young adults, familial lipoprotein lipase deficiency produces type I hyperlipoproteinemia, in which only serum chylomicron levels are elevated. It is not known for certain why the VLDL is not also raised, but it is likely that hepatic lipase can catabolize the lower levels of VLDL produced in childhood, although it

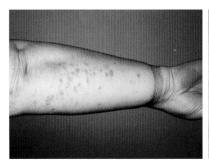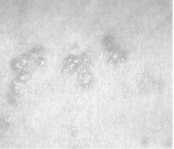

Figure 5.3 Eruptive xanthomata in a patient with severe (type V) hyperlipoproteinemia.

is unable to compensate for the absence of LPL as far as chylomicron catabolism is concerned. With advancing age, VLDL production increases to levels above those that can be cleared by lipoprotein lipase. As a result, VLDL and chylomicrons accumulate in the circulation, and type V hyperlipoproteinemia becomes apparent.

Physical signs. Eruptive xanthomata are characteristic of extreme hypertriglyceridemia. They appear as yellow papules on the extensor surfaces of the arms and legs, buttocks and back (Figure 5.3). Hepatosplenomegaly is common, and imaging shows the liver to be fatty. Bone-marrow biopsy may reveal foam cells. Because the triglyceride-rich lipoprotein may interfere with the determination of transaminases, giving spuriously high values, liver disease, in particular alcoholic liver disease, may be difficult to exclude other than by the prompt resolution of the syndrome when a low-fat diet is instituted. Other features include lipemia retinalis, with both the retinal veins and arteries appearing white (Figure 5.4).

Atheroma is not a complication of familial lipoprotein lipase deficiency, but it does complicate severe hypertriglyceridemia in which there is LPL activity, albeit diminished. It is difficult to make a precise estimate of the risk from the hyperlipidemia because it is so commonly associated with insulin resistance or frank diabetes, which are themselves risk factors for atherosclerosis. If these are included as part of the syndrome, both CHD and peripheral arterial disease are common.

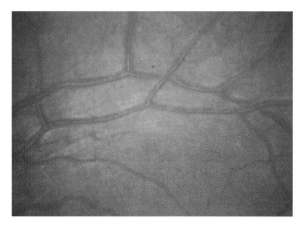

Figure 5.4 Lipemia retinalis. Reproduced courtesy of Dr JP Miller, University Hospital of South Manchester, UK.

The reason why the complete absence of LPL removes the risk of atheroma is not known with certainty. It may be because:

- the incidence of diabetes is not increased in familial lipoprotein lipase deficiency
- fibrinogen and factor VII activity are not increased
- the conversion of VLDL and chylomicrons to the atherogenic intermediate-density lipoprotein (IDL) and remnant lipoproteins, respectively, is impaired in the absence of LPL
- serum LDL and apoB levels are often normal or decreased in familial lipoprotein lipase deficiency, any increase in serum cholesterol being due to the cholesterol in VLDL and chylomicrons.

Acute pancreatitis may occur when serum triglyceride levels exceed 20–30 mmol/L (1800–2700 mg/dL). The presentation of acute pancreatitis is similar to that arising from other causes. However, increased serum amylase activity may not be present. Falsely low values may result from interference by triglyceride-rich lipoproteins in the laboratory method. All laboratories should inspect serum for milkiness (see Figure 5.2) before reporting normal or only moderately raised serum amylase activity in patients with severe abdominal pain. Clinicians may otherwise wrongly exclude the diagnosis of acute pancreatitis in favor, for example, of perforated peptic ulcer. Some patients do not develop acute pancreatitis, even when serum triglyceride levels exceed 100 mmol/L (9000 mg/dL). Others may experience recurring acute episodes.

Chronic pancreatitis does not occur – generally the pain subsides within a few hours or days of starting nasogastric aspiration and intravenous fluids (with nothing being taken by mouth). Pseudocysts develop occasionally if treatment is delayed.

Recurrent abdominal pain, not typical of pancreatitis, sometimes occurs in patients prone to marked hypertriglyceridemia. It may mimic irritable bowel syndrome. Severe abdominal pain may also be the result of splenic infarction.

Pseudohyponatremia is another complication of extreme hyper-triglyceridemia, and may lead to serious consequences if unrecognized. In pseudohyponatremia, spuriously low serum sodium values are reported because much of the volume of the serum aliquot on which the sodium measurement is made is occupied by lipoproteins rather than water. When the serum triglycerides exceed 40–50 mmol/L (3600–4500 mg/dL), the concentration of sodium in the aqueous phase (and thus the serum osmolality) may be normal, while spurious serum sodium levels of 120–130 mmol/L are reported. The hazard is that these will be misinterpreted by the clinician, and a patient already seriously ill with pancreatitis, or occasionally uncontrolled diabetes, will be made more so by infusion of large volumes of isotonic saline or, worse, hypertonic saline.

Focal neurological syndromes such as hemiparesis, memory loss and loss of mental concentration may complicate extreme hypertriglyceridemia; cerebral ischemia may result from a sluggish microcirculation caused by the high concentrations of chylomicrons in the blood. Paresthesias, particularly in the feet, may also be an occasional feature, even in the absence of diabetes. Sicca syndrome and polyarthritis have also been described, but undoubtedly the most common articular association is with gout (see page 83).

Dietary modification. For patients with serum triglyceride levels exceeding 10 mmol/L (900 mg/dL), fat intake of any type must be limited; chylomicrons persisting in the fasting state will be contributing to the hypertriglyceridemia, and these are formed from any kind of dietary fat. For patients with hypertriglyceridemia prone to pancreatitis or with eruptive xanthomata and hepatosplenomegaly, restriction of daily fat intake to 20 g or below may be necessary. Medium-chain triglycerides and fish oil are of no value in this situation. Carbohydrate and proteins must be substituted for fat in patients who are not obese. A dietitian attached to a specialized unit is usually best placed to give this type of advice and training.

Drug therapy is generally less effective than a low-fat diet in severe hypertriglyceridemia. Fibrates or nicotinic acid can, however, be of value.

Hypertriglyceridemia – Key points

- Severe hypertriglyceridemia increases the risk of pancreatitis, not coronary heart disease.
- Moderate hypertriglyceridemia with elevated apoB markedly increases the risk of coronary heart disease. Statins are the first-line therapy to reduce the risk of coronary heart disease in these patients.

Key references

Brunzell JD. Familial lipoprotein lipase deficiency and other causes of chylomicronemia syndrome. In: Scriver CR et al., eds. *The Metabolic and Molecular Bases of Inherited Disease*, 7th edn, vol 2. New York: McGraw Hill, 1995:1913–32.

Durrington PN. Hyper-triglyceridaemia. In: *Hyperlipidaemia, Diagnosis and Management*, 2nd edn. Oxford: Butterworth-Heinemann, 1995:190–214.

Durrington PN. Triglycerides are more important than epidemiology has suggested. *Atherosclerosis* 1998;141(suppl 1):S57–62.

Type III hyperlipoproteinemia has several synonyms:
- broad β disease
- floating β disease
- dysbetalipoproteinemia
- remnant removal disease.

It is rare, probably affecting fewer than 1 in 5000 people, and rarer still in premenopausal women and children. Type III hyperlipoproteinemia has the distinction of being the first clinical syndrome to be associated with primary hyperlipoproteinemia, and was described by Addison (who also described adrenal insufficiency and pernicious anemia) and Gull (physician to Queen Victoria) in 1851.

The condition is due to the presence of increased amounts of chylomicron remnants and IDL (or partially metabolized VLDL), often collectively termed β-VLDL, in the circulation. This is the result of decreased clearance of these lipoproteins at the apoE (or hepatic remnant) receptor.

Type III hyperlipoproteinemia undoubtedly causes accelerated atherosclerosis in the coronary, iliac, femoral and tibial arteries. Intermittent claudication occurs at least as frequently as CHD, and the incidence of the latter is about the same as that in FH. In FH, peripheral arterial disease is uncommon relative to the frequency of CHD, indicating that the atherogenic process in the leg arteries is much more susceptible to the larger lipoprotein particles in type III hyperlipoproteinemia than to the smaller LDL particles in FH.

Underlying mechanism

Type III hyperlipoproteinemia is generally an autosomal-recessive condition with variable penetrance. A mutation or polymorphism of the apoE gene appears to occur in all cases, and this impairs the binding of apoE to its receptor. A polymorphism, apoE2, in which cysteine is substituted for arginine at position 158 (Figure 6.1), is the most

65

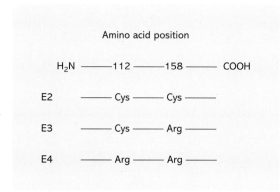

Figure 6.1 Amino-acid substitutions in the commonly occurring genetic polymorphisms of apoE. Cys, cysteine; Arg, arginine.

common genetic association. At least 90% of patients with type III hyperlipoproteinemia are homozygous for apoE2.

More often than not, however, apoE2 homozygosity, which is present in around 1% of the population, does not itself impose such a severe strain on lipoprotein metabolism that hyperlipoproteinemia develops; its combination with some other disorder that causes overproduction of VLDL or some additional catabolic defect is required. This explains the association of type III hyperlipoproteinemia with diabetes and hypothyroidism. More often, the additional stimulus to hyperlipoproteinemia is obesity or the co-inheritance of a polygenic tendency to hypertriglyceridemia. Rarer mutations of apoE have been described, including a mutation leading to apoE deficiency. These mutations behave similarly to apoE2 homozygosity clinically, although they may not require other factors for the expression of the type III phenotype. Heterozygous apoE deficiency finds little clinical expression but, interestingly, mutations directly involving the receptor-binding domain of apoE (amino acids 124–150) produce the type III phenotype even in heterozygotes (dominant expression), implying that such mutations are a greater handicap to receptor clearance than mutations in which one gene does not produce apoE.

Diagnosis

Cholesterol and triglycerides. Serum cholesterol and fasting triglyceride concentrations are increased – typically to 7–12 mmol/L (280–480 mg/dL) for cholesterol and 5–20 mmol/L (450–1800 mg/dL) for triglycerides. The molar concentrations of cholesterol and triglycerides are often similar, and this may be a clue that a patient has type III hyperlipoproteinemia. Occasionally the condition is associated with marked hypertriglyceridemia because of overwhelming chylomicronemia.

Xanthomata are present in more than half of the patients with the type III lipoprotein phenotype. Striate palmar xanthomata (Figure 6.2) and tubero-eruptive xanthomata (Figure 6.3) are characteristic. Striate palmar xanthomata can simply be an orange discoloration of the palmar skin creases. They may, however, be more florid and appear as raised, seed-like lesions (sometimes even larger) in the skin creases of the palms, fingers and flexor surfaces of the wrists. Tubero-eruptive xanthomata occur over the elbows and knees, and sometimes over other tuberosities, such as the heels and dorsum of the interphalangeal joints of the fingers. They resolve entirely with successful treatment.

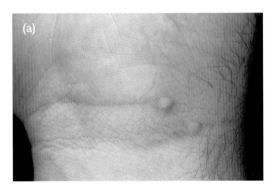

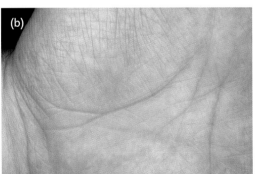

Figure 6.2 Striate palmar xanthomata (a) with some raised lesions, and (b) showing simply as an orange-yellow discoloration within the creases of the palm skin.

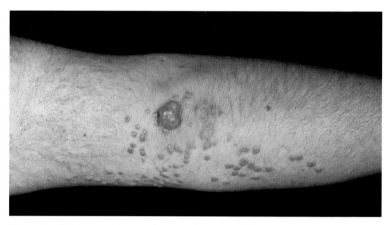

Figure 6.3 Tubero-eruptive xanthomata showing cauliflower-like tuberose deposits on the point of the elbow and eruptive satellite lesions.

Laboratory tests. The diagnosis of type III hyperlipoproteinemia is not difficult in the presence of typical xanthomata. When these are absent, laboratory tests are required. Type IIb or V hyperlipoproteinemia can give similar serum lipid levels.

Lipoprotein electrophoresis is still available in some hospital laboratories and, when it clearly shows separate pre-β (VLDL) and β (LDL) bands, is useful in differentiating type IIb from type III hyperlipoproteinemia. Often, however, the classical broad β band associated with type III hyperlipoproteinemia cannot be distinguished from the smear stretching from the origin into the pre-β and sometimes β regions in more severe cases of the type IIb or type V phenotype.

Polyacrylamide gel isoelectric focusing or DNA testing by restriction-fragment-length polymorphism, available in many specialized centers, can be used to identify apoE2 homozygosity. ApoE2 homozygosity in the presence of hyperlipidemia makes the diagnosis of type III virtually certain. When the apoE2 homozygosity is absent in a patient with the typical type III clinical phenotype, some other apoE mutation is usually present. Its identification, though of great theoretical value at a specialized center, is often impossible and, fortunately, is of little practical importance.

Testing for the apoE genotype may reveal that a patient does not have type III hyperlipoproteinemia, but provides the unwelcome finding that apoE4 is present. This mutation has been linked with Alzheimer's disease – certainly in its late-onset form but also, in some studies, with the early-onset type. It is probably wise for the laboratory reporting the apoE genotype results to report only whether apoE2 homozygosity is present or absent. Otherwise, information about many people's apoE4 genotype will be gratuitously available in their medical records without their consent or any explanation to them as to the possible consequences of its knowledge.

Ultracentrifugation. If clinical diagnosis of type III hyperlipoproteinemia requires confirmation in the absence of apoE2 homozygosity, plasma should be sent to a center that can identify cholesterol-rich VLDL (β-VLDL) typical of type III using ultracentrifugation.

It is also important to exclude paraproteinemia by immunoglobulin electrophoresis. This can produce hyperlipoproteinemia mimicking type III.

Treatment

Diet. Type III hyperlipioproteinemia can be responsive to a reduction in obesity. In the occasional lean patient, a diet in which monounsaturated and polyunsaturated fats and carbohydrates are substituted for saturated fat can be helpful unless triglycerides exceed 10 mmol/L (900 mg/dL). If this is the case, a diet low in all types of fat, with carbohydrate substitution, may be necessary.

Fibrates. Type III is also generally responsive to fibrate drugs, which should be regarded as the first-line treatment option. If after dietary modification the triglycerides remain only moderately elevated and cholesterol is in the normal range, it is generally wise to introduce fibrate therapy, because even a moderate increase in triglycerides probably indicates that the abnormal β-VLDL is present in quantities that may still be harmful.

Type III hyperlipoproteinemia – Key points

- Peripheral vascular disease is as common as coronary heart disease in these patients.
- Palmar and tubero-eruptive xanthomata are a key to diagnosis.
- Cholesterol and triglycerides are elevated, their molar concentrations often being similar.
- Fibrates are the first line of pharmacological therapy.

Key references

Mahley RW, Rall SC. Type III hyperlipoproteinemia (dysbetalipoproteinemia): the role of apolipoprotein E in normal and abnormal lipoprotein metabolism. In: Scriver CR et al., eds. *Metabolic and Molecular Bases of Inherited Disease.* New York: McGraw Hill, 1995:1953–80.

National Institute on Ageing. The Alzheimer's Association Working Group. Apolipoprotein E genotyping in Alzheimer's disease. *Lancet* 1996;347:1091–5.

Hyperlipidemia commonly coexists with other diseases. These diseases may be the complications of the hyperlipidemia, such as ischemic heart disease or pancreatitis. Sometimes, however, it is the hyperlipidemia which is the complication of another disease. In this case, the dyslipidemia represents a secondary rather than a primary derangement of lipoprotein metabolism. Hyperlipidemia may also be associated with another disorder more commonly than would be expected by chance alone, such as gout, even though no metabolic links are known between one and the other.

The secondary hyperlipidemias (Table 7.1) are important because:
- the secondary hyperlipidemia may be a cause of morbidity
- the hyperlipidemia may accelerate the progress of the primary disease, as has been suggested to be the case in renal and liver disease.

Table 7.2 shows the effect of some secondary hyperlipidemias on serum lipoprotein levels.

Diabetes mellitus

For far too long, diabetologists have been guilty of regarding diabetes mellitus as simply a disorder of carbohydrate metabolism, and insulin as involved only in maintaining euglycemia. These concepts were never sustainable. Diabetic ketoacidosis, after all, is the consequence of abnormal fatty acid metabolism. Even so, most physicians think of the coronary disease in diabetes as being the consequence of hyperglycemia. There is good reason to go beyond that view.

It is well documented, but not widely appreciated, that the incidence of microvascular disease differs little in diabetes around the world. By contrast, the incidence of macrovascular disease differs considerably, being much higher in societies in which a high proportion of energy comes from dietary fat rather than carbohydrate. Differences in prevalence of atherogenic dyslipidemias most likely explain these marked differences in coronary risk. The success of statin therapy in

TABLE 7.1

Diseases and physiological or pharmacological perturbations associated with secondary hyperlipidemia

Endocrine
- Diabetes mellitus
- Thyroid disease
- Pituitary disease
- Pregnancy

Renal disease
- Nephrotic syndrome
- Chronic renal failure

Drugs
- β-blockers
- Thiazide diuretics
- Steroid hormones
- Microsomal enzyme-inducing agents (e.g. phenytoin, phenobarbitone, griseofulvin)
- Retinoic acid derivatives (e.g. isotretinoin)
- HIV retroviral therapy

Hepatic disease
- Cholestasis
- Hepatocellular disease
- Cholelithiasis

Immunoglobulin excess
- Myeloma
- Macroglobulinemia
- Systemic lupus erythematosus

Hyperuricemia

Miscellaneous
- Glycogen storage disease
- Lipodystrophies

Nutritional
- Obesity
- Alcohol
- Anorexia nervosa

reducing clinical events and death in patients with type 2 diabetes provides indisputable support for the importance of LDL particle number in the pathogenesis of vascular disease in these patients.

Hypertriglyceridemia is the dominant hyperlipidemia in diabetes. Moderately raised triglyceride levels are common, and occasionally severe hypertriglyceridemia occurs, sometimes to levels in excess of 100 mmol/L (9000 mg/dL), leading to the development of eruptive xanthomata and occasionally other features of the chylomicronemia syndrome. Lipemia retinalis can interfere with laser photocoagulation therapy for diabetic retinopathy. Lipoprotein lipase is activated by insulin. Thus its activity is diminished with insulin deficiency and/or resistance associated with uncontrolled diabetes. There is generally an additional fault in triglyceride metabolism, predisposing to hypertriglyceridemia, for severe hypertriglyceridemia to occur: often this is a mutation in one of the lipoprotein lipase genes, leading to a defect in triglyceride catabolism which in the absence of diabetes may have produced only a modest rise in triglycerides. Less often, tubero-eruptive xanthomata and striate palmar xanthomata indicate that florid type III hyperlipoproteinemia has occurred in a genetically susceptible individual (usually an apoE2 homozygote).

In most patients whose diabetes is under reasonable glycemic control, any persisting hypertriglyceridemia is not due to a major defect in triglyceride catabolism, but to overproduction of VLDL by the liver. NEFA arriving at the liver from the adipose tissue and skeletal muscle in increased quantities are likely to be a major reason for increased

TABLE 7.2

Effect of some secondary hyperlipidemias on serum lipoprotein levels

Cause	VLDL	LDL	HDL
Type 1 diabetes	↑	– or ↓	– or ↑
Type 2 diabetes	↑↑	↑	↓
Hypothyroidism	↑	↑↑	↑
Pregnancy	↑	↑	↑
Obesity	↑	– or ↑	↓
Alcohol	↑	– or ↑	↑
Nephrotic syndrome	↑	↑↑	– or ↓
Chronic renal failure	↑	–	↓
Cholestasis	–	↑↑ (LpX)	↓
Hepatocellular disease	↑ (IDL)	–	↓
Hyperuricemia	↑	–	↓

IDL, intermediate density lipoprotein;
LpX, lipoprotein X

hepatic triglyceride synthesis and VLDL secretion. NEFA are released in increased quantities from adipose tissue when the quantity of adipose tissue is increased (i.e. in obesity), which often occurs in type 2 diabetes mellitus. Added to this, the enzyme within adipocytes that hydrolyzes their stored triglyceride to produce glycerol and NEFA – hormone-sensitive lipase – is regulated by insulin. Insulin inhibits intracellular hormone-sensitive lipase, but activates LPL. Therefore, in insulin resistance, the hormone-sensitive lipase becomes active, and increased amounts of free fatty acids (FFA) are released from adipose tissues. At the same time, triglyceride clearance from the circulation may be diminished by the lowered activation of LPL.

In diabetes, triglyceride release from the liver is further facilitated by decreased insulin secretion and/or insulin resistance, which will decrease the direct inhibitory effect of insulin on the secretion of VLDL by hepatocytes. Even in insulin-treated diabetes, the liver is likely to remain deficient in insulin because insulin administered via the subcutaneous route arrives at the liver from the systemic circulation rather than via the portal vein: physiologically, the concentration of insulin in the portal circulation is several times that in the systemic circulation. To achieve such high portal insulin levels by systemic administration of insulin would subject peripheral tissues to grossly supraphysiological levels.

Patients with type 1 diabetes mellitus are less likely to have hypertriglyceridemia than those with type 2 diabetes. This may be partly because insulin therapy is the rule in type 1 diabetes, and also because other factors predisposing to hypertriglyceridemia, such as obesity, and β-blocker and diuretic therapies, are more common in type 2 diabetes. There may, however, be a more fundamental reason. FFA are disposed of by the liver in three major processes:
• complete oxidation
• partial oxidation (ketogenesis)
• esterification (triglyceride synthesis).
When hepatic energy requirements are met, only ketogenesis and esterifiction are possible. In type 2 diabetes, NEFA are not readily converted to ketone bodies, whereas in type 1 diabetes their entry into the mitochondria, where β-oxidation occurs, is facilitated for reasons

not entirely understood. Resistance to ketogenesis in type 2 may thus carry with it a predisposition to hypertriglyceridemia.

Even minor elevations of triglycerides indicate increased CHD risk in diabetic populations. Low HDL cholesterol levels often coexist with hypertriglyceridemia, particularly in type 2 diabetes. In patients destined to develop type 2 diabetes, raised serum triglycerides and low HDL often precede the onset of glycemia by many years. Those patients yet to develop glycemia of diabetic proportions will have insulin resistance. It is not certain to what extent the insulin resistance syndrome is really pre-diabetes.

The atherogenicity of hypertriglyceridemia in diabetes is unlikely to involve directly the triglyceride-rich lipoproteins that are responsible for the elevated serum triglyceride levels. Rather it is likely to result from smaller, lipid-poor lipoproteins produced by their catabolism. There is evidence that increased quantities of small, dense LDL are produced in type 2 diabetes with hypertriglyceridemia at least partly due to an increase in CETP activity, which also contributes to the low HDL cholesterol. Also, in both types of diabetes, remnant particles or IDL probably persist at higher concentrations than in non-diabetics. There may also be a defect in the regulation of postprandial lipoprotein metabolism in diabetes. Normally the insulin secreted when the products of digestion enter the circulation inhibits hepatic VLDL secretion and promotes hepatic triglyceride storage at a time when triglyceride-rich lipoprotein production is high. This relieves pressure on the triglyceride catabolic pathways, such as those involving LPL and the apoE receptor, preventing the accumulation of remnants and IDL in the circulation postprandially. Later, when insulin levels decline, hepatic VLDL secretion increases and stored triglycerides are mobilized. In diabetes, failure to suppress VLDL secretion following meals occurs because of insulin resistance or deficiency, leading to high levels of remnant particles and IDL in the circulation.

Serum LDL cholesterol and apoB levels. Typical results for a group of 249 adult subjects with type 2 diabetes are shown in Table 7.3, which lists the average levels for each parameter as well as the percentile of the population with which the value accords. It is evident that total and

TABLE 7.3

Lipid and apoB levels in type 2 diabetic patients (n = 249)

	Mean value	Percentile of normal population
Age	59 years	
Total serum cholesterol	5.34 mmol/L (205 mg/dL)	~ 50th
Total serum triglycerides	2.13 mmol/L (189 mg/dL)	~ 60th
LDL cholesterol	3.28 mmol/L (126 mg/dL)	~ 50th
apoB	114 mg/dL	~ 70th
HDL cholesterol	1.12 mmol/L (43 mg/dL)	~ 35th

From Sniderman AD et al. *Diabetes Care* 2002;25:579–82

LDL cholesterol are normal, triglycerides elevated and HDL cholesterol decreased. The level of small, dense LDL is elevated also. Note that the apoB is high (70th percentile) compared with the LDL cholesterol (50th percentile). Figure 7.1 shows two ways of dividing the overall group into phenotypes: the first based on triglyceride and LDL cholesterol, the second on triglyceride and apoB. Note that in the first, only about 20% of patients have an elevated LDL cholesterol. By contrast, about 40% have elevated LDL particle number based on apoB. Even though apoB testing is not available to most clinicians, knowledge of the underlying increase in apoB, small, dense LDL and IDL helps to explain the benefit of statin and fibrate therapy in diabetes evident in the studies HPS, 4S, CARE, LIPID and VAHIT.

Serum HDL cholesterol concentrations tend to be low in type 2 diabetes, whereas in type 1 they are normal or even raised. The low levels in type 2 diabetes are largely explained by the presence of associated hypertriglyceridemia, obesity, cigarette smoking, abstention from alcohol, raised CETP activity and low LPL activity and the use of drugs such as β-blockers. These factors are less common in type 1 diabetes, and some other influence – probably insulin therapy – tends to increase HDL. A possible mechanism is that insulin increases HDL as a result of stimulating LPL activity. The raised HDL cholesterol in type 1 diabetes is not as protective against atheroma as would be expected in non-diabetics, probably because it has a diminished capacity to protect LDL against oxidative modification.

Effect of drugs. Oral hypoglycemic agents do not adversely affect lipoprotein levels in therapeutic trials, and improvements in glycemic control may even produce some improvement in lipid profiles.

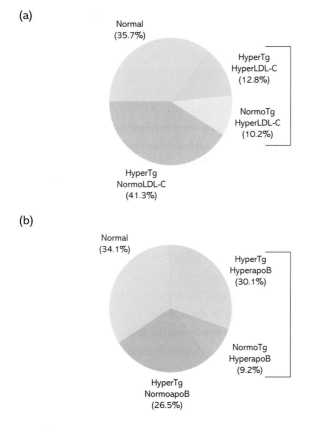

(a)

Normal
(35.7%)

HyperTg
HyperLDL-C
(12.8%)

NormoTg
HyperLDL-C
(10.2%)

HyperTg
NormoLDL-C
(41.3%)

(b)

Normal
(34.1%)

HyperTg
HyperapoB
(30.1%)

NormoTg
HyperapoB
(9.2%)

HyperTg
NormoapoB
(26.5%)

Figure 7.1 Two ways of dividing a group of 249 type 2 diabetic patients into lipid-level phenotypes: (a) based on serum triglyceride (Tg) and low-density lipoprotein cholesterol (LDL-C); (b) based on serum triglycerides and apolipoprotein B (apoB). Only 23% have elevated LDL cholesterol, but 39% have elevated apoB.

Metformin and guar gum also probably have an independent lipid-lowering action. Sadly, the use of sulfonylurea drugs in clinical practice is linked with decreased HDL and probably other adverse effects, such as increases in triglycerides and cholesterol. This is because the use of these drugs in practice is all too often associated with body weight gain. Insulin too, though its action is to lower triglycerides and cholesterol and raise HDL, may stimulate weight gain and thus increase insulin resistance, which will tend to nullify or even reverse any beneficial effects.

Proteinuria, hypertension and hyperfibrinogenemia often coexist with hyperlipidemia in diabetes and increase coronary risk considerably. Nephropathy, as in the case of primary renal disease, may influence lipoprotein metabolism. Proteinuria in diabetes indicates a generalized increase in vascular permeability, and thus macromolecules such as LDL may enter the arterial subintima at increased rates – an effect aided and abetted by hypertension.

Thyroid disease

Serum LDL cholesterol and, more rarely, serum triglycerides are raised in hypothyroidism. Receptor mediated LDL catabolism is decreased; triglyceride catabolism and LPL activity may also be reduced. HDL levels also tend to be increased because of diminished transfer of cholesteryl ester to other lipoproteins. These effects may be reversible with thyroxine replacement (Figure 7.2), which also restores biliary cholesterol excretion to normal where it was previously depressed.

Subclinical hypothyroidism – that is, raised serum thyroid-stimulating hormone (TSH) but thyroxine in the normal range – may influence serum LDL slightly. In one survey, raised serum TSH was present in 20% of women over the age of 40 years with serum cholesterol exceeding 8 mmol/L (320 mg/dL). Although only 5% were actually hypothyroid, findings such as these underline the importance of adequately excluding hypothyroidism in those with hypercholesterolemia beyond midlife.

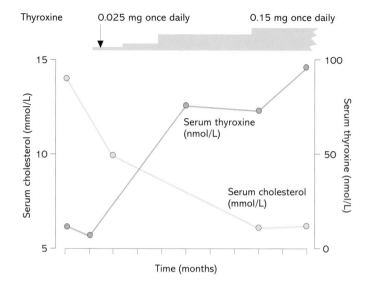

Figure 7.2 Effect of thyroxine-replacement therapy on serum cholesterol in a patient with hypothyroidism.

Hyperthyroidism. There is a tendency towards decreased LDL and HDL cholesterol in hyperthyroidism, but hypertriglyceridemia can occur.

Obesity

The overall relation of obesity to the risk of cardiovascular disease is not strong. However, if cases are divided into those with abdominal versus peripheral obesity, risk is high for the former but not for the latter. In both, insulin resistance is present. In abdominal obesity, hypertriglyceridemia with elevated apoB is frequent, whereas in peripheral obesity it is not.

Sex plays a major role in the pathophysiology of the two forms of obesity. Abdominal obesity is so common in males that the pattern is called android obesity. By contrast, peripheral obesity is common in females, and this pattern is designated gynoid obesity. Given that the omental depot constitutes such a small portion of the total amount of adipose tissue, it is still uncertain whether it is only the intra-abdominal adipose tissue that is responsible for the metabolic differences between the two obesity syndromes. It seems just as likely that female adipocytes, regardless of site, are better fatty-acid trappers than male adipocytes. In any case, it underlines the importance of sex hormones as determinants of adipose tissue function and therefore of the level of atherogenic lipoproteins in plasma.

Alcohol

Alcoholic beverages, particularly beer and wine, are energy rich and may be a cause of obesity. In addition, alcohol itself affects lipoprotein metabolism. Its dominant effect is to produce hypertriglyceridemia by increasing hepatic triglyceride synthesis. In turn, this leads to increased VLDL secretion. Fatty liver ensues if the mechanism for VLDL assembly and secretion fails to keep pace with production of triglyceride. Usually, alcohol overindulgence produces type IV hyperlipoproteinemia, but in individuals with a constitutional tendency to delayed triglyceride catabolism a spectacular type V hyperlipoproteinemia may occur; this may be one explanation for the association between alcohol consumption and acute pancreatitis. The increase in hepatic triglyceride synthesis stems partly from the ethanol-induced inhibition of oxidation of substrates other than itself. This tends to divert NEFA away from oxidative pathways into triglyceride synthesis. Triglyceride synthesis is further accelerated by the increased serum NEFA released from adipose tissue when ethanol is taken during fasting, or by the increase in food-induced fatty-acidemia caused by alcohol taken during a meal.

Serum LDL cholesterol levels tend to be low and HDL cholesterol raised in chronic alcoholics, unless liver disease has developed. The effect on HDL is evident in moderate drinkers, due predominantly to an effect on smaller HDL particles (HDL_3), whereas in heavy drinkers the measurably greater increase in HDL is due to the larger HDL_2.

Recognizing occult alcoholism is obviously important, particularly in hypertriglyceridemic patients prone to pancreatitis. Measuring serum γ-glutamyl transpeptidase is not always helpful in identifying patients who drink heavily, because it may be raised in patients with hypertriglyceridemia unrelated to alcohol.

Renal disease

Nephrotic syndrome. When proteinuria occurs in patients with relatively normal creatinine clearance, the predominant effect is to increase LDL (either from increased production of VLDL or by an increase in the amount of LDL directly secreted by the liver), thus producing hypercholesterolemia. The severity of the hypercholesterolemia is often proportional to the decrease in serum albumin.

Hypertriglyceridemia in nephrotic syndrome is unusual in the absence of hypercholesterolemia; it is more likely where chronic renal failure is also present, when it is often associated with decreased lipoprotein LPL. VLDL secretion by cultured hepatocytes decreases in response to albumin in the culture medium; the intravenous infusion of albumin or other macromolecules into patients with nephrotic syndrome reduces LDL levels. Both effects may be due to changes in osmotic pressure or to viscosity, as other macromolecules affect VLDL secretion in a similar way.

Serum HDL cholesterol levels are usually normal or decreased in nephrotic syndrome. Even when total HDL is normal, there is a shift towards smaller particles, so that the HDL_2 subfraction decreases while HDL_3 often increases. Loss of HDL from the circulation increases because of leakage from the kidney, and this is related to the selectivity and extent of the glomerular leak. Immunoreactive apolipoprotein AI in quantities equal to the normal daily apolipoprotein AI production may be found in the urine; to maintain relatively normal serum HDL cholesterol levels, HDL production is greatly increased in many patients with proteinuria.

Chronic renal failure without proteinemia. VLDL and LDL account for a higher proportion than normal of total serum triglyceride in patients with renal failure. There is also a tendency for remnant particles to persist in the circulation. The underlying cause is uncertain, but may relate to decreased activity of both LPL and hepatic lipase. Insulin resistance associated with renal failure does not appear to increase NEFA flux as it often does in other conditions. Hemodialysis further exacerbates hypertriglyceridemia; heparin depletes LPL and, in addition, there is loss of apolipoprotein CII, the activator of LPL, from

81

the circulation. Chronic ambulatory peritoneal dialysis leads to the absorption of considerable amounts of glucose from the peritoneum, producing obesity and exacerbating hypertriglyceridemia. In addition, LDL apoB is often raised, even when LDL cholesterol levels are not.

Serum HDL cholesterol levels are low in patients with chronic renal failure, while serum levels of lipoprotein (a) (Lp(a)) are often markedly elevated in all types of renal disease. Lp(a) comprises an LDL-like particle that contains apo(a) in addition to the usual apoB. Apo(a) is a member of the plasminogen supergene family and has much structural similarity with plasminogen. It appears to be an independent risk factor for CHD and cerebrovascular disease when it is present in high concentrations. Whether increased Lp(a) contributes to heightened susceptibility to atherosclerosis in renal disease is currently uncertain.

Many of the lipoprotein abnormalities resolve following renal transplantation, if good renal function is established. However, hyper-lipidemia persists in about one quarter of patients, perhaps because of corticosteroid therapy, weight gain, antihypertensive therapy and, possibly, ciclosporin treatment.

Liver disease

Cholestasis. Hypercholesterolemia occurs in obstructive jaundice without severe hepatocellular dysfunction. This is due to an increase in unesterified cholesterol in particles of hydrated density similar to that of LDL. Moderate hypertriglyceridemia and an increase in the plasma phospholipid lecithin (phosphatidylcholine) may also occur.

The lipoproteins of density similar to LDL are not true apoB-containing LDL, levels of which may be low, but are predominantly another lipoprotein designated lipoprotein X (LpX). This contains unesterified cholesterol and phospholipid in an approximately equal molar ratio. LpX has a lamellar structure and on electron microscopy appears as stacks of disk-like vesicles. LpX comprises 6% protein, of which at least half is albumin enclosed within the vesicles. Apolipoproteins, particularly apoC, are present on their surface. LpX migrates towards the cathode on electrophoresis on agar (but not agarose), which is unusual for a plasma lipoprotein. Biliary cholesterol does contribute to the cholesterol of LpX, but diversion of this from the obstructed biliary tree back into the circulation is, on its own, insufficient to explain the extent of hypercholesterolemia occurring in many patients. LCAT deficiency (see page 17) also contributes to the accumulation of unesterified cholesterol, but again this is unlikely to be the sole cause of the hypercholesterolemia, because only relatively small quantities of LpX are formed when LCAT activity is even more profoundly decreased in familial LCAT deficiency. In patients with biliary obstruction, LpX in the blood appears to be largely due to the reflux into the circulation of biliary phospholipids, which attract cholesterol out of cell membranes.

LpX is catabolized by the reticuloendothelial system, including Kupffer cells. Although it is not itself taken up by the hepatocyte, it may interfere with hepatic uptake of chylomicron remnants. The emerging view is that a system may exist for the sequestration of remnants in the space of Disse before uptake by the hepatocyte; it is interesting to speculate that this may be a site of their interaction with LpX. This may explain the persistence of remnant-like lipoproteins in patients with obstructive jaundice.

Hepatocellular disease is often accompanied by moderate hyper-triglyceridemia. This is due to triglyceride-rich lipoproteins with density in the VLDL and LDL range, which have, however, β-electrophoretic mobility, forming a broad β-band on electrophoresis. The HDL present also has β-mobility and, when isolated in the ultracentrifuge, consists predominantly of small particles. The accumulation of small HDL and the decrease in cholesteryl ester is secondary to LCAT deficiency, and the lipoproteins intermediate between VLDL and LDL probably build up because of hepatic lipase deficiency and other damage to the remnant-removal mechanism.

Hyperuricemia and gout

Hyperuricemia is present in a high proportion (probably half or more) of men with hypertriglyceridemia. As a result, gout commonly presents in patients with hypertriglyceridemia, particularly when hyperuricemia has been further 'precipitated' by thiazide diuretic administration. The reason for the association is not entirely clear, as it appears to be more common than might be explained by the frequent coincidence of factors, such as obesity and high alcohol consumption, with hypertriglyceridemia.

Hypertriglyceridemia and hyperuricemia are not causally related, as lowering uric acid with allopurinol does not affect triglyceride levels; conversely, with two exceptions, lipid-lowering drug therapy does not alter the serum urate concentration. The two exceptions are nicotinic acid, which raises urate, and fenofibrate, which lowers it. The latter effect, however, is not mediated through the triglyceride-lowering action of fenofibrate, but through an independent uricosuric effect. Both urate and triglyceride levels may decrease on a weight-reducing diet, suggesting that they may both be epiphenomena of some underlying nutritional process. It has been suggested that dietary carbohydrate is important. Dietary fructose, which is taken up almost exclusively by the liver, induces hypertriglyceridemia and also increases urate levels, probably by diverting energy away from the hepatic urate-scavenging pathway into fructose phosphorylation.

Drugs

A large number of drugs in common use affect serum lipoprotein concentrations (Table 7.4). Those most commonly encountered in the lipid clinic are diuretics and β-blockers.

Thiazide diuretics raise VLDL and LDL by mechanisms that have not been elucidated. Their effect is generally small, but it may be more substantial in diabetes, which they also exacerbate. Diuretics do not alter HDL levels.

β-blockers, regardless of cardioselectivity, tend to increase serum triglyceride concentrations by an effect on VLDL, and to decrease HDL cholesterol. There is no convincing evidence that they affect total cholesterol or LDL cholesterol. Their effect on serum triglycerides may be marked in patients with pre-existing hypertriglyceridemia. A decrease in the clearance of triglyceride-rich lipoproteins appears to be the mechanism, perhaps resulting from a direct effect reducing the activity of lipoprotein lipase, or from diversion of blood flow away from the vascular bed of muscle, one site rich in the enzyme.

TABLE 7.4

Drugs affecting lipoprotein metabolism

Drug	VLDL	LDL	HDL
Thiazides	↑	↑	–
β-blockers without ISA	↑	–	↓
Estrogens	↑	– or ↓*	↑
Progestogens	–	↑	↓
Androgens	↓	↑	↓
Glucocorticoids	– or ↑	↑	↑
Hepatic microsomal enzyme-inducing agents (e.g. phenobarbitone, rifampin, griseofulvin)	–†	–†	↑
Retinoic acid derivatives (e.g. isotretinoin)	↑	–	–

ISA, intrinsic sympathomimetic activity
*Decreased LDL in postmenopausal women
†May be unsustained increase

β-blockers with intrinsic sympathomimetic activity (ISA) have little or no effect on serum HDL and triglycerides. Of this class, pindolol has the highest ISA, but has found little favor as an antihypertensive and is unsuitable for the management of angina. Acebutolol and oxprenolol, with ISA about half that of pindolol, but about double those of other β-blockers, may be valuable in some patients with hypertriglyceridemia when β-blocker therapy cannot be avoided. Labetalol, which combines α- and β-blocking activity, is reported to have little effect on serum lipoproteins.

Many reports suggest that α-blockers, calcium-channel antagonist vasodilators, direct-acting vasodilators and angiotensin-converting enzyme inhibitors are either without effect on serum lipoproteins or may even have apparently favorable effects, such as raising HDL cholesterol. There is, however, no evidence as yet that pharmacologically induced changes of this type significantly alter disease morbidity or mortality.

Estrogens tend to raise the serum triglyceride level because of increased hepatic VLDL production. Occasionally their administration in women with pre-existing hypertriglyceridemia has led to gross hyperchylomicronemia and consequent acute pancreatitis. In most women, the increase in triglycerides is small. Paradoxically, improvement has been reported in women with type III hyperlipoproteinemia, possibly because estrogen induction of remnant receptors outweighs any deleterious effect of increased VLDL production.

Estrogens also raise serum HDL concentrations and, in post-menopausal women, decrease serum LDL levels. Although their effects may therefore appear beneficial, this idea must be treated with caution. First, because the opportunities to administer estrogen preparations alone are few, generally only postmenopausal women who have undergone hysterectomy can be considered. Estrogen must be combined with a progestogen for most women requiring it for contraception or as hormone-replacement therapy. The final balance of favorable and unfavorable effects on lipid metabolism in any individual will then depend on the preparation used. Second, estrogens increase the risk of thromboembolism and, like other steroids, will have mineralocorticoid and glucocorticoid activity, thus increasing the tendency to hypertension and diabetes mellitus.

Androgens generally cause the opposite effects to those achieved with estrogens: a decrease in serum HDL cholesterol and VLDL and an increase in LDL.

Progestogens increase LDL and decrease HDL – the strength of the effect depends on their androgenicity.

HIV antiretroviral therapy commonly produces combined hyperlipidemia with an elevated apoB. This is due to increased VLDL secretion which, in turn, is the consequence of therapy-induced reduced fatty-acid-trapping capacity by adipose tissue. It is daunting to consider adding yet another medication – statins – to the already too long list of drug therapies these patients must consume. However, the better the prognosis becomes, the more important the issue, because there is no reason to believe the arteries of these patients will be immune to the effects of this potentially atherogenic dyslipoproteinemia.

Other drugs. Many drugs other than those discussed above affect lipoprotein metabolism (e.g. retinoic acid derivatives used in dermatology). Also important, because of the high rate of atherosclerosis in recipients of renal transplants, are the corticosteroids and ciclosporin used as immunosuppressive agents. Of great theoretical interest are drugs and chemicals that induce hepatic cytochrome P450, because of an associated increase in serum HDL levels. Such drugs include phenytoin, phenobarbitone, rifampin and griseofulvin. Chlorinated pesticides, such as lindane and DDT, have the same effect.

Secondary hyperlipidemia – Key points

- Dyslipidemias are often secondary to other diseases.
- Dyslipidemia is a major mechanism of vascular disease in type 2 diabetes mellitus.
- Statins are the first line of therapy for diabetic dyslipidaemias.
- Overall, hormone replacement therapy increases the risk of cardiovascular disease.

Key references

Baraona E, Lieber CS. Alcohol. In: Betteridge DJ et al., eds. *Lipoproteins in Health and Disease.* London: Arnold, 1999:1011–36.

Durrington PN. Secondary hyperlipidaemia. In: *Hyperlipidaemia, Diagnosis and Management.* Oxford: Butterworth-Heinemann, 1995:291–360.

Edwards CM, Stacpoole PW. Rare secondary dyslipidaemias. In: Betteridge DJ et al., eds. *Lipoproteins in Health and Disease.* London: Arnold, 1999:1069–98.

Kissebah AH, Krakower GR. Endocrine disorders. In: Betteridge DJ et al., eds. *Lipoproteins in Health and Disease.* London: Arnold, 1999:931–41.

Lean MEJ. Obesity and eating disorders. In: Betteridge DJ et al., eds. *Lipoproteins in Health and Disease.* London: Arnold, 1999:881–95.

Miller JP. Liver disease. In: Betteridge DJ et al., eds. *Lipoproteins in Health and Disease.* London: Arnold, 1999: 985–1009.

Muller-Wieland D, Krone W. Drug-induced effects. In: Betteridge DJ et al., eds. *Lipoproteins in Health and Disease.* London: Arnold, 1999:1037–48.

Short CD, Durrington PN. Renal disorders. In: Betteridge DJ et al., eds. *Lipoproteins in Health and Disease.* London: Arnold, 1999:943–66.

Sniderman AD, Scantlebury T, Cianflone K. Hypertriglyceridemic hyperapoB: the unappreciated atherogenic dyslipoproteinemia in type 2 diabetes mellitus. *Ann Intern Med* 2001;135:447–59.

Recent criticisms leveled at the effectiveness of dietary treatment mostly stem from overviews of the effect of diet on lowering serum cholesterol in clinical trials. There is no doubt that clinical trials of diet are difficult to design and execute. Nevertheless, in practice, some people achieve a worthwhile reduction in cholesterol with dietary advice, and it is cheap to implement in comparison with drug treatment.

Diet can decrease both cholesterol and triglyceride levels and can significantly improve glycemic control in diabetes, sometimes even rendering the patient non-diabetic. The overviews of trials in which CHD incidence was the outcome measure also show that CHD risk can be diminished with diet. The fear of those critical of dietary treatment is that it may be employed as a sole means of therapy in high-risk patients who might otherwise derive considerable benefit from drug therapy. Diet should therefore be regarded as an adjunct to lipid-lowering drug therapy in patients at high CHD risk, such as those with established CHD. It should be part of the general lifestyle advice given to lower-risk patients for whom lipid-lowering drug therapy is not justified (see Chapter 9).

Failure of dietary modification to decrease cholesterol below some arbitrary level is not in itself an indication for lipid-lowering drug therapy; generally the need for drug therapy is determined by CHD risk. It is sometimes questioned whether it is worth bothering with diet in high-risk patients when the statins, for example, can produce a much more substantial decrease in serum cholesterol. The reason for continuing to advocate dietary advice is that the decrease in CHD incidence in many dietary trials was apparently greater than would have been expected from the decrease in serum cholesterol achieved in the trials. It seems, therefore, that there may be some additional beneficial effects that patients relying exclusively on pharmacological measures are denied. Not to emphasize diet in CHD prevention is to broadcast the wrong message to the public and to those responsible for determining nutritional policy.

Dietary advice should be offered to most people whose serum cholesterol exceeds 5.0 mmol/L (200 mg/dL). General advice is probably of limited value if the cholesterol is substantially higher or there is concern about CHD risk. Referral to a dietitian or to a nurse who has trained in dietary counseling is then generally advisable. If the patient does not do the cooking in the household, then whoever does should also be present on such a visit. The importance of such a referral is that a personal dietary history will be taken so that advice can be tailored to the patient's own dietary preferences.

There are two essential components to dietary prevention of CHD: weight loss and reduction of saturated fat intake.

Weight reduction

Obesity is clearly related to hypercholesterolemia, hypertriglyceridemia, low HDL cholesterol (Figure 8.1), high blood pressure, insulin resistance and diabetes mellitus. The obese patient should be advised to lose weight. Even reduction of moderate obesity is sometimes helpful – all hyperlipidemias in the obese respond to weight reduction. Failure to lose weight complicates the management of hyperlipidemia, hypertension and diabetes. The best way to lose weight is to eat less, particularly fat. A consistent weight loss of about 1 lb/week (0.45 kg/week) is a very laudable target for weight reduction. Exercise cannot substitute for a reduced energy intake, except in unusual cases, but it may be critical in maintaining the decreased body weight achieved by dietary restriction. Claims that exercise alone can produce weight loss are generally based on calculations that neglect to subtract the energy expenditure of whatever else the patient would have been doing, had he or she not been exercising at the time.

Reducing saturated fat intake

The second important element of dietary modification involves decreasing saturated fat intake. Saturated fats in the diet increase both serum cholesterol and triglyceride levels; replacing them with carbohydrates (other than simple sugars and syrup), polyunsaturated fats or monounsaturated fats lowers the serum cholesterol and triglyceride levels. In the non-obese, in whom an energy deficit is not

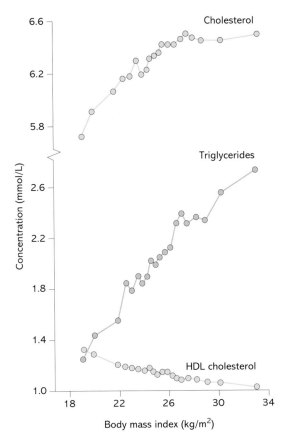

Figure 8.1 The effect of increasing degrees of obesity on serum lipids and HDL cholesterol. Reproduced, with permission from BMJ Publishing Group, from Thelle et al. *Br Heart J* 1983;49:205–13.

needed, a traditional north European and North American diet can be modified by:

- increasing the intake of potatoes, pulses, rice, pasta and fish
- using olive oil products, soybean, sunflower, safflower, corn or rapeseed (canola) oils.

Other dietary advice

Fruit and vegetables have a small effect in decreasing blood cholesterol in their own right because of their soluble fiber content. They can be

91

eaten freely because they do not contribute to obesity and can enhance the variety of a healthy diet enormously. They may even protect against CHD in other ways, for example by providing antioxidants and folic acid.

Fiber. There is probably no point in deliberately advising the consumption of high-fiber foods, particularly those rich in insoluble fiber. Wheat bran has no effect on blood cholesterol, and the so-called high-fiber diet has deterred many people from following a cholesterol-lowering diet.

Dietary cholesterol does not contribute greatly to blood cholesterol levels. It is probably wise to limit eggs to about three a week, but most patients can still enjoy avocado or shellfish when they get the chance. Foods are often labelled 'low in cholesterol'. This is unimportant. What is important is that they are 'low in saturated fat', if your patient is concerned with lowering blood cholesterol, and 'low in fat' if the patient is mainly trying to lose weight. Refined carbohydrate, such as sugar in drinks and confectionery, should be avoided if the patient is trying to lose weight. The less-refined carbohydrate foods, such as bread, rice and pasta, beans and potatoes, have a much lower energy content than fat, and their consumption should be encouraged (in moderation only for those trying to lose weight).

Coffee. There is probably no point in restricting coffee intake as a means of lowering blood cholesterol, because its effect is small.

Alcohol is not harmful to the heart in moderate amounts. However, in the obese it may be a major source of excess energy intake. In hyperlipidemia, particularly when associated with raised triglyceride levels, and in hypertension, it may be necessary to monitor a period of abstinence to assess the effects of alcohol.

Dietary treatment – Key points

- In the obese, dyslipidemic weight loss is the key strategy.
- Eating less works.
- Exercise is more helpful in maintaining weight loss than in achieving it.
- Alcohol is hypercaloric.

Key references

Durrington PN. Diet. In: *Hyperlipidaemia, Diagnosis and Management*. Oxford: Butterworth-Heinemann, 1995:225–57.

Grundy SM. Dietary therapy of hyperlipidaemia. *Baillieres Clin Endocrinol Metab* 1987;1:667–98.

Vascular disease, whether coronary, cerebral or peripheral, is an absolute indication for intensive dietary and pharmacological therapy, as are genetic hyperlipoproteinemias (e.g FH and Type III) and diabetes mellitus. For most other patients the decision to treat and the target for therapy are based on the total risk of disease. Different schemes have been presented to incorporate the risk due to age, blood lipids and blood pressure and the likelihood of a major clinical event calculated over usually a 10-year period. These are reviewed in Chapter 10. A major difficulty of a therapeutic target based on total serum or LDL cholesterol is that there is little evidence that on-treatment LDL cholesterol is predictive of outcome. By contrast, there is considerable evidence that on-treatment levels of apoB remain predictive, and therefore apoB-guided statin therapy should be much more effective than LDL-cholesterol-guided statin therapy when it becomes more widely available.

Statin secondary prevention trials

Five major trials – 4S, CARE, LIPID, GREACE, HPS – have been conducted using statins to reduce the risk of vascular events in patients with symptomatic vascular disease or at high risk of vascular disease. Cholesterol levels varied substantially, being highest in 4S and lowest in important subsets in HPS; levels in CARE and LIPID were intermediate.

The first of these landmark trials was the Scandinavian Simvastatin Survival Study (4S trial) in which simvastatin was administered to moderately hypercholesterolemic patients with known CHD. Total mortality was reduced as was the rate of coronary events. The Cholesterol and Recurrent Events (CARE) and the Long-term Intervention with Pravastatin in Ischemic Disease (LIPID) both tested the effects of pravastatin. In CARE, the sum of fatal and non-fatal coronary events was significantly reduced, while in LIPID, both total and coronary rates were reduced in the treated group compared with

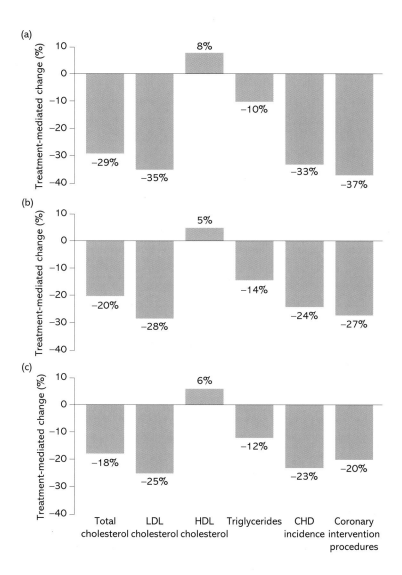

Figure 9.1 Results from three secondary prevention trials of statin therapy:
(a) the Scandinavian Simvastatin Survival Study (4S), (b) the Cholesterol and
Recurrent Events study (CARE) and (c) the Long-term Intervention with
Pravastatin in Ischemic Disease (LIPID) study. The mean total serum
cholesterol values at randomization were 6.7 mmol/L (260 mg/dL), 5.4 mmol/L
(209 mg/dL) and 5.6 mmol/L (216 mg/dL), respectively.

the placebo group. The results from the three trials are summarized in Figure 9.1.

The patients in the CARE and LIPID trials had total and LDL cholesterol levels that were lower than in 4S. In the CARE trial, all subjects had a total cholesterol below 6.0 mmol/L (240 mg/dL), with the average being 5.2 mmol/L (209 mg/dL). The average LDL cholesterol was reduced from 3.5 to 2.5 mmol/L (139 to 98 mg/dL). Although overall benefit was shown in the treated group in CARE, subgroup analysis showed no significant improvement in outcome for the treated group starting with an LDL cholesterol below 3.1 mmol/L (125 mg/dL). This subgroup analysis attracted considerable attention, particularly when it was tied to findings in an earlier coronary angiographic trial, the Harvard Reversibility Project (HARP), which also failed to show benefit from marked cholesterol lowering. However, with the completion of the GREek Atorvastatin and Coronary heart disease Evaluation (GREACE) study and the larger Heart Protection Study (HPS), it is obvious that the whole issue of LDL cholesterol targets must be thoroughly rethought (see Chapter 10).

Results of the GREACE, and HPS studies were published in 2002. Both of them provide further confirmation of the findings of the earlier trials and of the wisdom of having lower cholesterol threshold levels for the introduction of statin treatment in high-risk patients and having lower therapeutic target LDL levels.

In GREACE 1600 men and women aged < 70 years with established CHD were randomized to receive usual care or atorvastatin, 10–80 mg daily, with the aim of achieving LDL cholesterol levels of < 100 mg/dL (2.5 mmol/L) – the target recommended by the Third Adult Treatment Panel (ATPIII) of the National Cholesterol Education Program (NCEP) (see Chapter 10). Of the atorvastatin-treated patients, 95% achieved these LDL cholesterol levels, whereas only 3% of the usual-care group did. LDL cholesterol – which was initially on average 4.7 mmol/L (190 mg/dL), with total serum cholesterol 6.6 mmol/L (260 mg/dL) – was 41% lower in the atorvastatin-treated patients than in those receiving usual care at the end of the 3-year study (Figure 9.2). New CHD events were 51% lower in the atorvastatin group.

The Heart Protection Study. In HPS, 20 536 patients aged 40–80 years, whose serum cholesterol was ≥ 3.5 mmol/L (140 mg/dL), were randomized to receive simvastatin, 40 mg each evening, or placebo. Initially, on average, LDL cholesterol was 3.4 mmol/L (140 mg/dL) and total serum cholesterol was 5.9 mmol/L (240 mg/dL). At the end of the 5-year study, in the treated group, compared with the placebo group, LDL cholesterol was 29% lower; major vascular events (coronary, stroke and revascularization) were 25% fewer for patients with no CHD on entry, and were 24% fewer for those with CHD on entry (Figure 9.3). The decrease in relative risk was the same in patients with diabetes mellitus. It was also not significantly lower in patients with serum cholesterol < 5 mmol/L (200 mg/dL) than in those with higher values.

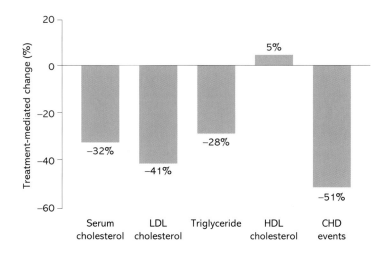

Figure 9.2 Results from the GREek Atorvastatin and Coronary heart disease Evaluation (GREACE) study showing changes in outcome measures over 3 years for the group receiving atorvastatin, 10–80 mg daily, relative to those for the group receiving usual care. Mean total serum cholesterol at randomization was 6.6 mmol/L (260 mg/dL). Only 3% of those receiving usual care achieved the ATPIII target for LDL cholesterol (< 100 mg/dL [2.5 mmol/L]), whereas 95% of the atorvastatin-treated group did so.

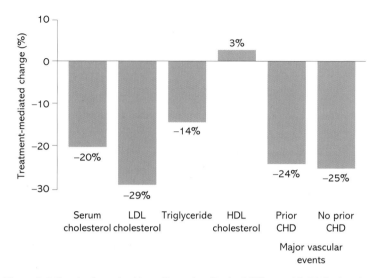

Figure 9.3 Results from the Heart Protection Study (HPS; n = 20 536) showing changes in outcome measures over 5 years for the group receiving simvastatin, 40 mg daily, relative to those for the placebo group. Mean total serum cholesterol at randomization was 5.9 mmol/L (240 mg/dL). The patients without previous CHD were at high risk on account of non-coronary atherosclerosis or diabetes and/or were men aged > 65 years with hypertension.

The HPS contained no strictly primary prevention group, because the patients without CHD at entry had cerebral or peripheral vascular disease or diabetes or were elderly men with hypertension. The annual vascular event rate in the group without CHD at entry thus exceeded that in the WOSCOPS or AFCAPS/TexCAPS studies (see next section). The HPS's major importance is that it confirms the view that the reduction in relative CHD risk with a particular dose of a particular statin is the same in all high-risk groups whether they be men or women, elderly or young, no matter whether the risk arises from pre-existing CHD, other atherosclerotic disease or by an adverse combination of risk factors including diabetes, hypertension and smoking. It also strongly suggests that there is no cholesterol threshold below which patients cannot benefit from statin therapy. The apparent contradictory finding in the smaller CARE study seems to have arisen because the study was statistically underpowered to detect a loss of statin effect, on account of the smaller number of patients with low initial cholesterol levels. HPS also showed that, in all the high-risk groups randomized, stroke risk was significantly reduced by 25%, consistent with a meta-analysis of 4S, CARE and LIPID and with findings in GREACE. This strongly suggests that prevention of stroke should be listed among the benefits of statin therapy.

Statin primary prevention studies

Fewer data are available for primary prevention studies with statins. Two major primary prevention studies have been completed: the West of Scotland Coronary Prevention Study (WOSCOPS) and the Air Force/Texas Coronary Atherosclerosis Prevention study (AFCAPS/TexCAPS) (Figure 9.4). WOSCOPS involved middle-aged moderately hypercholesterolemic men, many of whom were smokers. The trend to benefit was clear, with a significant reduction in the number of events, though not quite in mortality. In AFCAPS/TexCAPS, cholesterol levels were much lower than in WOSCOPS, but many subjects also had low HDL cholesterol levels. The degree of benefit in terms of relative risk reduction in AFCAPS/TexCAPS was similar to that achieved in the secondary prevention trials. The major difference was in the absolute number of events.

The most important risk factor for a coronary event is the presence of coronary disease. Patients with coronary disease are overwhelmingly likely to die from it. Therefore, in trials of secondary prevention, there will be lots of coronary events to prevent. The same is not the case for primary prevention, and one clear lesson from WOSCOPS and AFCAPS/TexCAPS is that lipid levels alone, except for those with extreme elevations, are relatively weak individual predictors of risk. Therefore, any prevention strategy either exclusively or primarily based on lipid levels will require a very large number of patients to be treated for any significant number to benefit. It is for this reason that calculation of absolute coronary risk is helpful in deciding whom to treat in primary prevention.

A number of cost–benefit studies have been published. Statin therapy is expensive, but the cost in relation to benefit diminishes as the risk of disease increases. In all these studies, yearly costs for treating one

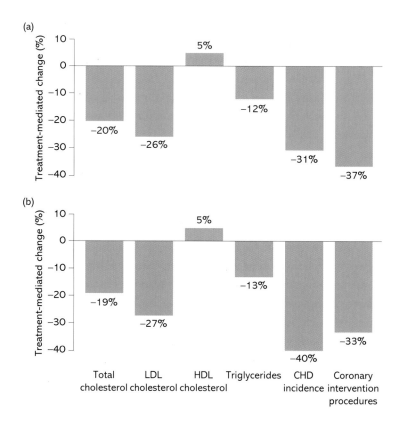

Figure 9.4 Results from the two primary prevention trials of statin therapy: (a) the West of Scotland Coronary Prevention Study (WOSCOPS), and (b) the Air Force/Texas Coronary Atherosclerosis Prevention Study (AFCAPS/TexCAPS). The mean total serum cholesterol values at randomization were 7.0 mmol/L (280 mg/dL) and 5.5 mmol/L (220 mg/dL), respectively.

individual are usually favorably compared with standardized costs for individuals with other problems, such as end-stage renal disease requiring hemodialysis. However, the number of these patients is orders of magnitude less than the number of patients who could benefit from statin therapy. Unfortunately, cost–benefit studies do not project total costs, just individual costs. The benefit of statin therapy clearly outweighs cost in secondary prevention and primary prevention in those whose CHD risk exceeds 20% in the next 10 years. As the cost of statins diminishes, lower levels of risk may justify treatment; they may already do so when treatment costs are borne by the patient. Benefit was shown in AFCAPS/TexCAPS when the annual CHD risk was only 1%. The decisions by consensus groups on when to recommend statin therapy are not determined solely by the scientific evidence but are heavily influenced by cost. Individuals may legitimately place a different value on their lives.

Limitations: what should the target of therapy be?

The major limitation of the clinical trials is our lack of knowledge as to what the target of statin therapy should be. Accordingly, we do not know the maximal benefit that could follow from their use. On average, clinical events are reduced by about one third or less in the primary and secondary prevention trials. But is that the maximum benefit achievable? ATPIII has recommended a target level of LDL cholesterol of 2.5 mmol/L (100 mg/dL). But there are several difficulties with that decision.

First, HPS demonstrated that statin treatment in high-risk subjects starting with target levels of LDL cholesterol achieved proportionately as much benefit as those with higher levels. That is to say, treating beyond that ATPIII target brought clinical benefit. Specifically, more than 6700 subjects in HPS had LDL cholesterol < 3.0 mmol/L (120 mg/dL) at the onset of the trial, whereas 3500 had values below 2.5 mmol/L (100 mg/dL), the current target level for ATPIII. Both these groups benefited proportionately just as much as those with higher levels at baseline. These findings are clearly at variance with the target levels chosen by ATPIII and the European consensus groups.

It is important to note that there is also considerable evidence in the previous trials questioning whether statin therapy should be guided by the levels of LDL cholesterol. Except in 4S, on-treatment levels of LDL cholesterol have had little or no predictive value in the major statin trials. That contrasts with apoB. On-treatment apoB was predictive in 4S, AFCAPS/TexCAPS, LIPID and the Leiden Heart Study as well as the report by Moss and his colleagues. Taken together, these studies constitute strong evidence of a linear relation between the level of apoB and residual risk in subjects being treated with statins. The results suggest that the clinical events could be reduced to a substantially greater extent if statin therapy were guided by levels of apoB rather than by the levels of LDL cholesterol. An apoB target level of < 90 mg/dL has been accepted by the Canadian Cardiovascular Society. As more data become available, the target may be lowered.

Fibrate trials

The statin trials have yielded consistent, straightforward results. That has not been the case for the fibrate trials. The WHO/Clofibrate trial was the first in the series and produced an unhappy result in that total deaths during the trial and 1 year after ending it were significantly higher in the clofibrate group than in the control group. A different fibrate, gemfibrozil, was tested in the Helsinki Heart Study. Although there was a significant reduction in combined cardiac endpoints in this primary prevention trial of hyperlipidemic men, the death rate was again higher in the treated group, although this time not significantly so.

Two major fibrate secondary prevention trials have been reported: VA-HIT and the Bezafibrate Infarction Prevention Study (BIP). IN VA-HIT, which is the most positive of the fibrate trials, the subjects were, on average, 64 years old and all had a history of coronary disease. Gemfibrozil was administered to the 1264 men in the treated group and their outcome was compared with that in 1267 men in the placebo group over a mean follow-up of 5.1 years. Total and coronary death did not differ significantly, but therapy was associated with a significant reduction in a combined endpoint of coronary death and non-fatal myocardial infarction (22% vs 17.3%, $p < 0.06$). Benefit was related statistically to a small increase in HDL cholesterol, but not to the much larger drop in triglycerides. It is, of course, possible that benefit could be the consequence of a change in LDL composition. That is to say, several studies have shown that reduction in triglycerides results in a shift from the more atherogenic, small, dense LDL particles, which so regularly accompany hypertriglyceridemia, to the less atherogenic, normal, cholesterol-replete LDL particles.

In the BIP secondary prevention trial, 1548 patients received bezafibrate, a second-generation fibrate, and 1542 patients formed the

placebo group. Follow-up was for a mean of 6.2 years. There were
unfortunately many difficulties with the conduct of this study, including
a high use of additional lipid-lowering medications in both the placebo
and treatment group. In the event, there was no evidence of significant
clinical benefit in any of the parameters that were studied. There was a
significant reduction in clinical events in the subgroup with baseline
triglycerides > 200 mg/dL (2.2 mmol/L), but the groups were small and
the analysis was not prespecified.

Because hypertriglyceridemia and low HDL cholesterol are so
common in type 2 diabetes, fibrates have been commonly used in these
patients. There is some evidence supporting this view. Thus, subgroup
analysis of the patients with type 2 diabetes in the VA-HIT trial did
show significant reduction of combined cardiovascular endpoints.
Similarly, the DAIS trial demonstrated significantly less angiographic
progression of coronary lesions in patients with type 2 diabetes given
bezafibrate. There was also a trend to fewer clinical events, but the trial
was much too small for the result to be significant. Taken together, the
evidence for fibrates as first-line therapy in patients with or at high risk
of vascular disease is not convincing, and the results contrast markedly
with the uninterrupted series of successes obtained with statins,
although it must be admitted that our information about the benefits of
statins when triglycerides exceed 4.5 mmol/L (400 mg/dL) is limited. It
remains possible that fibrates may benefit patients with type 2 diabetes,
but they should probably only be considered as initial drug therapy
when triglycerides exceed 10 mmol/L (900 mg/dL) and then because of
their greater clinical efficacy in lowering triglycerides. There is a case
for combining them with statin therapy in particularly high-risk
patients when triglycerides exceed 2.2 mmol/L (200 mg/dL) despite
statin therapy, because they can decrease CHD risk in people with
elevated triglycerides – albeit a finding in patients not already receiving
statins. There is a risk of myositis about which patients should be
advised and monitored. Omega–3 fatty acids in the form of Omacor in
doses of around 4 g daily can decrease triglycerides by as much as
fibrates do, and they may be safer in combination with statins. They
were shown in the GISSI trial in doses of only 1 g to decrease coronary
events, particularly sudden cardiac death.

Guidelines

Generating national and multinational medical guidelines has become an enormous growth industry. These attempts at educating and advising physicians are important and necessary exercises. However, scientific rigor may occasionally play second fiddle to the necessity for consensus and, perhaps even worse, simplification by the expert for the non-expert. Statements of the highest importance may suddenly appear without any link to evidence. Nevertheless, there is an encouraging tendency, particularly apparent in recent guidelines such as those jointly agreed by the British Cardiac Society, British Hyperlipidaemia Association and British Hypertension Society, to take a more inclusive and balanced approach to risk-factor analysis, considering evidence in the widest context. This is crucial for primary prevention because plasma lipid values, except when extreme, are only crude and weak indicators of risk.

Hypertension, diabetes, smoking, male gender and family history are important risk factors. So is android obesity. Age becomes an ever more dominant risk factor as the decades pass. These risk factors may be thought of as either affecting LDL or affecting the interaction of LDL with the arterial wall, as is discussed in Chapter 2. A relatively low level of LDL cholesterol may justify treatment in a patient with a particularly adverse combination of these other risk factors, whereas substantially higher levels of LDL cholesterol may not do so in the absence of these other risk factors. An important exception to this is FH, where the natural history of the condition dictates that statin treatment is generally started in men at least by their early twenties and women by their mid-thirties. More nebulous but potentially important clinical syndromes, such as familial combined hyperlipidemia, can also guide prognosis and treatment.

Pharmacotherapy

Diet almost always precedes pharmacological therapy in the advocated regimens. Unfortunately, dietary therapy is rarely more than partially successful, and the reality for most individuals is that medication is required to achieve major changes in plasma lipoprotein levels. However impressive the safety record to date, lipid-lowering pharmacological therapy potentially carries some risk, which should never be overlooked. Moreover, the costs of therapy are substantial. They include not only the costs of the medication, but all the associated costs, such as laboratory, medical and nursing resources. But the costs go even further. There is loss of time from work to attend clinics and there is often an increase in absenteeism in those labeled with diagnoses of chronic medical conditions. That said, in those who can benefit, pharmacological therapy is well justified.

Statins inhibit HMG-CoA reductase, the enzyme which is physiologically rate-limiting for cholesterol biosynthesis. Their principal effect is to lower plasma LDL (both LDL cholesterol and particle number), although modest increases in HDL cholesterol and, depending on the agent and dose, variable decreases in plasma triglycerides also result. Postprandial remnant clearance may also be improved in some patients.

By altering the balance of cholesterol and cholesteryl ester within the hepatocyte, statins increase the removal of IDL and LDL, and decrease the production of VLDL and LDL. Although a number of non-lipoprotein effects have been reported, such as a decrease in platelet aggregability and decreased smooth-muscle cell proliferation within the arterial wall, the effects on the plasma lipoproteins – in particular the marked decrease in LDL – would appear to be the major mechanisms underlying clinical benefit.

On the basis of the evidence from clinical and angiographic studies, statins should be regarded as first-line therapy for patients with atherosclerotic vascular disease. The currently available agents differ somewhat in their pharmacological properties and potency. Most often used as monotherapy, statins have been used in combination regimens when LDL levels are particularly high and sometimes when it is necessary to lower both LDL and triglycerides. Addition of bile-acid sequestrants will result in further lowering of LDL without any increase in the risk of statin side-effects. This combination can be unsuitable where a clinically significant increase in triglycerides as well as LDL cholesterol persists after statin therapy has been introduced, because hypertriglyceridemia is often exacerbated by bile-acid-sequestrating agents.

For this reason, notwithstanding the slight increase in the risk of toxicity, statins have also been combined with fibrates, particularly in patients with familial combined hyperlipidemia, in order to reduce triglycerides more profoundly and to increase HDL cholesterol more markedly. This regimen will also alter LDL composition so that a smaller proportion of the more atherogenic, small, dense LDL particles will persist. A newer combination therapy for combined hyperlipidemia has been omega–3 fatty acids and statins – good results have been reported.

The statins currently available are atorvastatin, fluvastatin, lovastatin, pravastatin and simvastatin. All are of proven efficacy in lowering LDL cholesterol. Lovastatin (not available in the UK), pravastatin, simvastatin and atorvastatin have been shown in clinical trials to decrease CHD risk. Thus, if the clinician were to practice strictly evidence-based medicine, these drugs should be employed in the doses used in the trials with coronary events as end points (that is, lovastatin, 20–40 mg, pravastatin, 40 mg, simvastatin, 10–40 mg, or atorvastatin, 10–80 mg, daily). To employ different doses of these drugs or to use the other statins is to extrapolate from clinical trials and to regard the coronary prevention action of the statins as a class effect. Although this may be attractive on the grounds of cost, such a view may be premature. In patients with high CHD risk whose LDL levels are not satisfactorily controlled or who are intolerant of evidence-based doses of statins, different dosages or the use of newer potent statins may be particularly justified. This rationale will hold for the newest of the statins, rosuvastatin, which seems likely to be available in the near future.

Side-effects. About 1% of patients have a substantial (more than threefold), persistent but asymptomatic elevation of hepatic transaminase levels. The effect is usually dose related. Therapy may be continued in the face of mild increases in enzyme levels, although substantial increases call for discontinuation. Following normalization of hepatic function, re-institution of treatment at lower doses of a different statin should be considered. Hepatic enzyme levels should be measured 6 and 12 weeks after starting therapy, and semiannually thereafter.

Asymptomatic elevation of creatine kinase, muscle weakness, pain or stiffness may occur. More rarely, frank rhabdomyolysis with acute renal failure may result, usually when statins have been given in combination with other hypolipidemic agents, such as fibrates or nicotinic acid, or concurrently with agents such as ciclosporin in heart and renal transplant patients. The frequency of severe adverse reactions in these circumstances is happily much lower than was originally believed, and combination therapy may be used with caution in fully informed, frequently monitored patients. There is also a risk of myositis in patients on statin therapy when antibiotics such as erythromycin are administered. Such combinations should be avoided.

Levels of creatine kinase reaching two or three times the upper limit of laboratory reference ranges are not uncommon in patients not receiving lipid-lowering therapy. Sometimes these can be linked to bouts of muscular exertion. The clinician should be aware that such increases can occur spontaneously and are not necessarily the result of statin therapy. Furthermore, muscular ache, particularly in the shoulders and neck, is a common phenomenon that can lead to inappropriate discontinuation or rejection of statin therapy.

Although the evidence is incomplete, some experimental data suggest that statins have a teratogenic effect; administration during pregnancy, therefore, is inadvisable. On the other hand, there is no evidence of mutagenic effects.

As with any class of drugs, a range of side-effects such as headache, nausea, non-specific skeletomuscular symptoms and tiredness may be reported with statins. In placebo-controlled trials, these have not been reported with a substantially greater frequency in treated groups than in placebo groups. Nevertheless, they are the most commonly reported side-effects. Changing to another statin agent is often helpful.

Fibrates generally have a much weaker effect on LDL cholesterol levels than do statins. Indeed, there may be an increase in LDL cholesterol concentration with these agents in patients with raised triglycerides and relatively low LDL cholesterol levels at the outset of treatment. They are effective in decreasing the circulating concentration of small, dense

LDL, although the clinician is not in a position to assess this effect from routinely available lipid measurements.

The mechanism of action of fibrates is not well understood, but may include decreased triglyceride production by the liver and improved triglyceride clearance by peripheral tissues. The most important clinical effects are a marked reduction in serum triglycerides and an increase in HDL cholesterol. Depending on the agent and the type of hyperlipidemia, LDL cholesterol and apoB levels may be reduced, but not usually by more than 10–20%. Postprandial triglyceride clearance is also improved after fibrate therapy.

Fibrates are certainly the pharmacological agents of choice in individuals with markedly elevated triglyceride levels and who are therefore at risk of pancreatitis. Normalization of plasma lipids also frequently occurs in patients with type III hyperlipoproteinemia. In other patients with vascular disease, lack of trial data demonstrating clinical efficacy means statin treatment should be first-line therapy. It is possible that in subgroups such as those with diabetes, fibrates may bring particular benefit given the characteristic lipid profile of hypertriglyceridemia, low HDL cholesterol and small, dense LDL in these patients, but again this awaits confirmation.

Side-effects are generally mild. Headache, gastrointestinal upset, rashes and pruritus have been reported. Mild elevations of hepatic and muscle enzymes may occur. Bile-acid lithogenicity is probably increased, at least in the early stages of treatment. Fibrates should be avoided in patients known to have gallstones, although only clofibrate has been shown in clinical trials to increase the incidence of clinically significant cholelithiasis.

Fibrates may interact significantly with anticoagulants such as warfarin, and great care should be exercised in their introduction in patients receiving such therapy. Their use should be avoided in patients with renal disease (bezafibrate, in particular, raises creatinine levels) and may cause a paradoxical rise in cholesterol in patients with cholestatic liver disease, in whom they are contraindicated.

Bile-acid resins. The currently available agents are non-absorbable anion exchange resins that bind bile salts irreversibly. The resulting depletion in the bile-acid pool leads to greater breakdown of cholesterol to form bile acids. In turn, this leads to upregulation of LDL receptors to maintain the cholesterol pool within the liver, and lowering of LDL levels typically by 10–20% (more in compliant patients). Plasma triglyceride levels, however, may increase substantially, particularly in those with already elevated values.

The major indication for these agents is in combination with a statin in patients with very high LDL levels. Under these circumstances, benefit can often be achieved with smaller, more acceptable daily doses (cholestyramine, 4–8 g; colestipol, 5–10 g). Stool softeners can be considered. There is an increased likelihood of gallstones developing with bile-acid sequestrants, although this may be lower in patients already receiving statins. Bile-acid sequestrants can decrease serum folate levels, and folate supplementation should be considered in vulnerable groups such as children and women who may become pregnant. In the Lipid Research Clinics Trial, cholestyramine decreased CHD incidence, and both cholestyramine and colestipol have been used either alone or in combination with other drugs in successful coronary angiographic regression trials. Evidence that they significantly decrease all-cause mortality is not available, however, and it is unlikely that further trials will be undertaken to test this.

Side-effects. Constipation, bloating and heartburn are the principal side-effects and are commonly encountered, limiting the usefulness of this class.

Nicotinic acid is a B vitamin that, in pharmacological doses (up to 7 g daily), markedly reduces VLDL and LDL and substantially increases HDL. It alone among the hypolipidemic agents may reduce Lp(a). Its mechanism of action is not certain, but involves reducing VLDL secretion by the liver, perhaps in response to reduced fatty acid release by adipocytes.

The advantages of nicotinic acid are that it improves the whole lipo-protein profile, and its cost is low. Opinions are divided about whether the dose should be taken all at once with the evening meal, allowing flushing (see below) to be endured in the privacy of one's own home, or whether it should be taken in divided doses to try to minimize side-

---

Drug treatment – Key points

- Statins reduce coronary heart disease and cerebrovascular disease events by about one third in both primary and secondary prevention.
- Evidence of clinical benefit is clear for statins but not yet unequivocal for fibrates.
- Much controversy remains as to what the targets of statin therapy should be. Our view of the evidence is that lower is better and that therapy guided by the apoB level will be more effective than that guided by LDL cholesterol level.

---

effects. In either case, it is customary to begin with 50 mg daily, working up to a dose of 3000 mg or above. The dose should be taken at the end of a meal with a small dose of aspirin at the beginning. Lipoprotein levels should be assessed 1 month later.

Side-effects limit its use. Flushing is virtually universal. It can be reduced if a small dose of aspirin or another prostaglandin inhibitor is taken shortly before nicotinic acid. More serious side-effects include gastritis and peptic ulcer exacerbation, hepatitis, gout and hyperglycemia. Significant interaction with statins can occur to produce rhabdomyolysis and renal failure.

Analogues and slow-release preparations. Because of its attractive effect on the lipoprotein profile, numerous attempts have been made to produce analogues or preparations of nicotinic acid that overcome the flushing problems. In many cases, these have simply made the flushing reaction unpredictable. Acipimox does appear to induce less flushing, but while it retains the triglyceride-lowering action of its parent nicotinic acid, it is much less effective at lowering serum cholesterol.

Ezetimibe is an intestinal cholesterol absorption inhibitor which interrupts the enterohepatic circulation of cholesterol and the absorption of dietary cholesterol. It lowers serum cholesterol by approximately 20%, an effect which is additive to the cholesterol-lowering effect of statins and has also been recorded in patients with homozygous FH. It may therefore prove to be an important adjunct to statin treatment for hypercholesterolemia.

Key references

Athyros VG, Papageorgiou AA, Mercouris BR et al. Treatment with atorvastatin to the National Cholesterol Education Program goal versus 'usual' care in secondary coronary heart disease prevention. The GREek Atorvastatin and Coronary-heart-disease Evaluation (GREACE) study. *Curr Med Res Opin* 2002;18:220–8.

Ballantyne CM, Herd JA, Dunn JK et al. Effects of lipid-lowering therapy on progression of coronary and carotid artery disease. *Curr Opin Lipidol* 1997;8:354–61.

DAIS. Effect of fenofibrate on progression of coronary-artery disease in type 2 diabetes: the Diabetes Atherosclerosis Intervention Study, a randomised study. *Lancet* 2001;357:905–10.

Downs JR, Clearfield M, Weis S et al. Primary prevention of acute coronary events with lovastatin in men and women with average cholesterol levels. Results of AFCAPS/TexCAPS. *JAMA* 1998;279:1615–22.

Durrington PN, Bhatnagar D, Mackness MI et al. An omega-3 polyunsaturated fatty acid concentrate administered for one year decreased triglycerides in simvastatin treated patients with coronary heart disease and persisting hypertriglyceridaemia. *Heart* 2001;85:544–8.

Frick MH, Elo H, Haapa K et al. Helsinki Heart Study: primary-prevention trial with gemfibrozil in middle-aged men with dyslipidemia. Safety of treatment, changes in risk factors, and incidence of coronary heart disease. *N Engl J Med* 1987;317:1237–45.

GISSI-Prevenzione Investigators. Dietary supplementation with n-3 polyunsaturated fatty acids and vitamin E after myocardial infarction: results of the GISSI-Prevenzione trial. *Lancet* 1999;354:447–55.

HARP. Effect of combination therapy with lipid-reducing drugs in patients with coronary heart disease and "normal" cholesterol levels. A randomized, placebo-controlled trial. Harvard Atherosclerosis Reversibility Project (HARP) Study Group. *Ann Intern Med* 1996;125:529–40.

Heart Protection Study Collaborative Group. MRC/BHF Heart Protection Study of cholesterol lowering with simvastatin in 20 536 high-risk individuals: a randomised placebo-controlled trial. *Lancet* 2002;360: 7–22.

Moss AJ, Goldstein RE, Marder VJ et al. Thrombogenic factors and recurrent coronary events. *Circulation* 1999;99:2517–22.

Oliver MF, Heady JA, Morris JN et al. A co-operative trial in the primary prevention of ischaemic heart disease using clofibrate: a report from the Committee of Principal Investigators. *Br Heart J* 1978; 40:106–18.

Roeters van Lennep JE, Westerveld HT, Roeters van Lennep HWO et al. Apolipoprotein concentrations during treatment and recurrent coronary artery disease events. *Arterioscler Thromb Vasc Biol* 2000;20:2408–13.

Rubins HB, Rubins SJ, Collins D et al. Gemfibrozil for the secondary prevention of coronary heart disease in men with low levels of high-density lipoprotein cholesterol. *N Engl J Med* 1999;341:410–18.

Sacks FM, Pfeffer MA, Moye LA et al. The effect of pravastatin on coronary events after myocardial infarction in patients with average cholesterol levels. *N Engl J Med* 1996;335:1001–9.

Scandinavian Simvastatin Survival Study Group. Randomised trial of cholesterol lowering in 4444 patients with coronary heart disease; the Scandinavian Survival Study. *Lancet* 1994;344:1383–9.

Shepherd J, Cobbe SM, Ford I et al., for the West of Scotland Coronary Prevention Study Group. Prevention of coronary heart disease with pravastatin in men with hypercholesterolemia. *N Engl J Med* 1995;333:1301–7.

The BIP Study Group. Secondary prevention by raising HDL cholesterol and reducing triglycerides in patients with coronary artery disease. The Bezafibrate Infarction Prevention (BIP) Study. *Circulation* 2000;102:21–7.

The Lipid Research Clinics Program. The Lipid Research Clinics Coronary Primary Prevention Trial. Results I: Reduction in incidence of coronary heart disease. *JAMA* 1984;251: 351–64.

The Long-Term Intervention with Pravastatin in Ischemic Heart Disease (LIPID) Study Group. Prevention of cardiovascular events and death with pravastatin in patients with coronary heart disease and a broad range of initial cholesterol levels. *N Engl J Med* 1998;339:1349–57.

Physicians now have an unparalleled opportunity to prevent vascular disease – but only if we act. We divide prevention strategies into those that apply to everyone and those that are necessary for selected groups. A healthy diet – a diet that is energy neutral for the patient who is not obese and energy negative for one who is, and that is not fatty acid excessive – is the most neglected but the most powerful act of prevention. Promoting exercise is wonderful not only for health, but also for self-esteem. Helping patients to stop smoking is critical. These are the fundamentals to prevent vascular disease, and they apply to everyone, but unfortunately most clinicians are better at listing them than implementing them.

However, there are also substantial numbers at high individual risk who need to be considered for pharmacological as well as dietary therapy. In almost all instances, this will mean statin therapy. Because vascular disease is so common and because pharmacological therapy remains expensive, deciding where to draw the line is a major social consideration. Medical experts have accepted this argument and have drawn up protocols to determine whether pharmacological therapy is justified. A positive decision is based on either clinical indication or the total risk profile.

Indications for pharmacological therapy based on clinical evidence of disease

There are two such indications.

- The first is objective evidence of vascular disease. This includes any evidence of coronary disease, cerebrovascular or peripheral vascular disease. In addition to symptoms, ECG and angiographic evidence, this would include, in our judgment, ultrasound evidence of disease in either the extracranial cerebral or peripheral vessels.
- The second absolute clinical indication in North America is diabetes, either type 1 or type 2. In type 1 diabetes, however, it remains unclear at what age hypolipidemic therapy should start.

Indications for pharmacological therapy based on risk assessment

The importance of identifying presymptomatic individuals who will develop early and accelerated vascular disease has led to the development of numerous guidelines around the world. From this complex process, an overall consensus is gradually starting to emerge. The recent ATPIII guidelines base the decision to treat on the overall risk rather than just the level of cholesterol. In this regard, the American approach now resembles that previously taken in Europe. Nevertheless, important differences remain between the American and European approaches, and so each is briefly summarized below.

The ATPIII approach. The approach of the Third Adult Treatment Panel (ATPIII) of the National Cholesterol Education Program (NCEP) is summarized in Figure 10.1. A target level of LDL cholesterol of 2.5 mmol/L (100 mg/dL) has been set for those with vascular disease, diabetes, or an estimated risk of a major event of > 20% over a 10-year period. For those with ≥ 2 risk factors, risk needs to be calculated from the Framingham tables. These are summarized in Tables 10.1 (males) and 10.2 (females). In the group with intermediate risk (10–20% chance of CHD over 10 years), the target LDL cholesterol is < 3.3 mmol/L (130 mg/dL). Similarly, in the group with low risk (< 10% chance of CHD over 10 years) and LDL cholesterol > 4.0 mmol/L (160 mg/dL), the target LDL cholesterol is also < 3.3 mmol/L (130 mg/dL). For those with < 2 risk factors, 10-year risk is not calculated, but if LDL cholesterol is > 4.8 mmol/L (190 mg/dL), it should be reduced with either dietary or drug therapy to < 4.0 mmol/L (160 mg/dL).

This is a more comprehensive approach, and we agree with this change in direction. However, there are a number of limitations that should be noted, as follows.

- The multiple groups and targets almost certainly will be confusing for practitioners.
- Risk due to lipids is calculated on the basis of total and HDL cholesterol, whereas the targets for therapy are levels of LDL cholesterol.

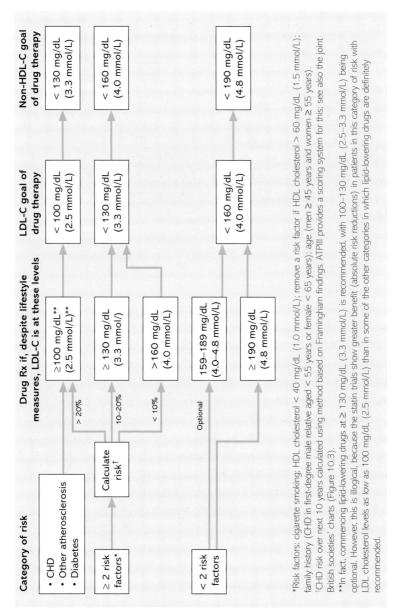

Figure 10.1 Synopsis of the Third Report of the National Cholesterol Education Program (NCEP) Expert Panel on Detection, Evaluation and Treatment of High Blood Cholesterol in Adults (Adult Treatment Panel III). Source: National Cholesterol Education Program 2001.

115

- The target levels are not evidence based – that is, they are not based on the results of clinical trials. Indeed the Heart Protection Study has shown that proportionately just as much benefit from statin therapy can be obtained in high-risk subjects who start with an LDL cholesterol of 2.5 mmol/L (100 mg/dL) as those who had much higher levels initially. This strongly suggests that an LDL cholesterol of 2.5 mmol/L (100 mg/dL) is not the right target level.

- The risk estimates are not valid for patients with FH, type III hyperlipoproteinemia or renal disease. These patients must be treated vigorously at whatever age they present. Type 1 diabetes is also a special case because these patients tend to have relatively high levels of HDL cholesterol but do not enjoy any protection against coronary disease. In these patients, we suggest using the total cholesterol alone and assuming an HDL cholesterol of 1.0 mmol/L (40 mg/dL).

- Hypertriglyceridemia remains a problem because it is not included as such in the ATPIII guidelines. As we have noted, hypertriglyceridemia is common in coronary patients. ATPIII does acknowledge the issue by producing a definition of the metabolic syndrome (Table 10.3). For these patients, it is suggested that risk and adequacy of therapy be gauged by non-HDL cholesterol, creating yet another number to remember and monitor.

The European approach is more conservative than that of the USA with respect to primary prevention. It is accepted that CHD, other major atherosclerosis, and familial hypercholesterolemia or other genetic hyperlipidemia call for statin therapy if serum cholesterol persists at ≥ 5 mmol/L (200 mg/dL) or LDL cholesterol at ≥ 3 mmol/L (120 mg/dL). It is recommended that in all other patients a calculation of risk based on Framingham results be made to assist the clinician in deciding who should receive lipid-lowering drug therapy. Currently the joint European cardiovascular societies' recommendations are being revised. Thus far, diabetes mellitus alone has not been accepted as a coronary risk equivalent unless proteinuria is present. The existing recommendations include a chart for the calculation of CHD risk which omits HDL cholesterol and is thus inaccurate. Also the threshold for the introduction of lipid-lowering drug therapy is 20% risk over 10 years, which recent clinical trials would indicate is too high.

The more recent recommendations of the joint British societies (JBS) (Figure 10.2) are probably therefore closer to what is acceptable practice in Europe. These provide a CHD risk chart which includes HDL cholesterol (Figure 10.3), and make a CHD risk of 15% over 10 years the indication for lipid-lowering therapy in primary prevention, if serum cholesterol is persistently ≥ 5 mmol/L (200 mg/dL) or LDL cholesterol ≥ 3 mmol/L (120 mg/dL). This is the same cholesterol threshold as for secondary prevention. Both primary and secondary prevention also have the same target serum and LDL cholesterol values in Europe. In the case of the UK, these are a serum cholesterol < 5 mmol/L (200 mg/dL) or a reduction of 25%, whichever gives the lower target. Equivalent LDL targets are LDL cholesterol < 3 mmol/L (120 mg/dL) or a reduction by 30%, whichever gives the lower target. The percentage reductions as well as absolute targets are included for patients whose pretreatment serum cholesterol or LDL cholesterol may be close to 5 or 3 mmol/L, respectively. It seems likely that, with the new trial evidence from GREACE and HPS, the ATPIII target for secondary prevention will eventually become the target universally adopted both for primary and secondary prevention – i.e. LDL cholesterol < 2.5 mmol/L (100 mg/dL) – and that diabetes mellitus will be more widely treated without resort to CHD risk calculation.

The JBS charts (like the Framingham risk equation) will underestimate risk if there is an adverse family history of premature CHD (female first-degree relatives aged < 65 years and male first-degree relatives aged < 55 years). Multiplying the risk shown on the chart by 1.5 is suggested in such circumstances. They will also underestimate risk in certain ethnic groups such as migrants from the Indian subcontinent, patients whose treated blood pressure values are used in the calculation, women with premature menopause, people with raised triglycerides, and people with impaired fasting glucose (6.0–6.9 mmol/L). In these cases clinical judgment must be used to adjust the calculated risk upwards. An alternative to the use of the JBS charts is to use the Framingham risk equation programmed into a computer or calculator. The Joint British Societies Cardiac Risk Assessor Programme, which

TABLE 10.1

Method of estimating 10-year risk of CHD for men
(Framingham point scores) provided in ATPIII*

Age (years)	Points
20–34	–9
35–39	–4
40–44	0
45–49	3
50–54	6
55–59	8
60–64	10
65–69	11
70–74	12
75–79	13

Total cholesterol (mg/dL)	Points				
	Age 20–39 years	Age 40–49 years	Age 50–59 years	Age 60–69 years	Age 70–79 years
<160	0	0	0	0	0
160–199	4	3	2	1	0
200–239	7	5	3	1	0
240–279	9	6	4	2	1
≥ 280	11	8	5	3	1

Smoking	Points				
	Age 20–39 years	Age 40–49 years	Age 50–59 years	Age 60–69 years	Age 70–79 years
Non-smoker	0	0	0	0	0
Smoker	8	5	3	1	1

TABLE 10.1 (CONTINUED)

HDL (mg/dL)	Points
≥ 60	−1
50–59	0
40–49	1
< 40	2

Systolic BP (mmHg)	If untreated	If treated
< 120	0	0
120–129	1	3
130–139	2	4
140–159	3	5
≥ 160	4	6

Point total	10-year risk (%)
< 9	< 1
9	1
10	1
11	1
12	1
13	2
14	2
15	3
16	4
17	5
18	6
19	8
20	11
21	14
22	17
23	22
24	27
≥ 25	≥ 30

* Third Report of the National Cholesterol Education Program (NCEP) Expert Panel on Detection, Evaluation and Treatment of High Blood Cholesterol in Adults (Adult Treatment Panel III) 2001

TABLE 10.2

Method of estimating 10-year risk of CHD for women (Framingham point scores) provided in ATPIII*

Age (years)	Points
20–34	–7
35–39	–3
40–44	0
45–49	3
50–54	6
55–59	8
60–64	10
65–69	12
70–74	14
75–79	16

Total cholesterol (mg/dL)	Points				
	Age 20–39 years	Age 40–49 years	Age 50–59 years	Age 60–69 years	Age 70–79 years
< 160	0	0	0	0	0
160–199	4	3	2	1	1
200–239	8	6	4	2	1
240–279	11	8	5	3	2
≥ 280	13	10	7	4	2

Smoking	Points				
	Age 20–39 years	Age 40–49 years	Age 50–59 years	Age 60–69 years	Age 70–79 years
Non-smoker	0	0	0	0	0
Smoker	9	7	4	2	1

TABLE 10.2 (CONTINUED)

HDL (mg/dL)	Points
≥ 60	−1
50–59	0
40–49	1
< 40	2

Systolic BP (mmHg)	If untreated	If treated
< 120	0	0
120–129	0	1
130–139	1	2
140–159	1	2
≥ 160	2	3

Point total	10-year risk (%)
< 0	< 1
0	1
1	1
2	1
3	1
4	1
5	2
6	2
7	3
8	4
9	5
10	6
11	8
12	10
13	12
14	16
15	20
16	25
≥ 17	≥ 30

* Third Report of the National Cholesterol Education Program (NCEP) Expert Panel on Detection, Evaluation and Treatment of High Blood Cholesterol in Adults (Adult Treatment Panel III) 2001

TABLE 10.3

Metabolic syndrome defined in ATPIII*

1. Abdominal obesity: waist circumference
   - Men: > 40 inch (102 cm)
   - Women: > 35 inch (88 cm)
2. Serum triglycerides ≥ 150 mg/dL (1.7 mmol/L)
3. HDL cholesterol
   - Men: < 40 mg/dL (1.0 mmol/L)
   - Women: < 50 mg/dL (1.3 mmol/L)
4. Blood pressure ≥ 130 / > 85 mmHg
5. Fasting glucose ≥ 110 mg/dL (6.1 mmol/L)

*Third Report of the National Cholesterol Education Program (NCEP) Expert Panel on Detection, Evaluation and Treatment of High Blood Cholesterol in Adults (Adult Treatment Panel III) 2001

can be downloaded from several websites, including www.medicine.man.ac.uk/stopmed, is an example of this. The program has the advantage that it gives stroke as well as CHD risk for both systolic and diastolic blood pressures.

Although we have provided in this book both the ATPIII scoring system and the British charts for CHD risk assessment, we do not recommend that they be used interchangeably with the guidelines for which they were not designed. The risk predicted by the two methods is slightly different, and the thresholds for intervention are therefore specific to the risk prediction method.

Risk calculation period. A limitation common to all recommendations based on absolute cardiovascular risk should be noted. That is, how artificial a 10-year span to calculate risk can be. Why should a man of 40 with a calculated risk just under that mandating therapy wait until he is 50, giving disease 10 more years to develop in his arteries, before therapy can begin? We know coronary disease begins in the teens and may be well advanced anatomically by the twenties and thirties. It just takes a while longer for clinical expression. The fact of the matter is

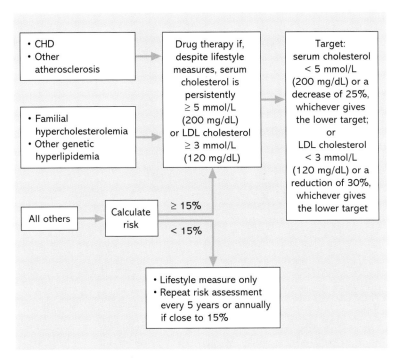

Figure 10.2 The joint British societies' (JBS) recommendations for cholesterol-lowering treatment to prevent CHD. CHD risk over next 10 years is calculated using a method based on Framingham findings, such as the JBS chart (Figure 10.3). Currently, as an interim measure where resources are limited, the National Health Service permits a CHD risk ≥ 30% over 10 years for the introduction of statin therapy as the minimum level of care. Joint European recommendations suggest ≥ 20% over 10 years. Source: Working Party of the British Cardiac Society, British Hyperlipidaemia Association and British Hypertension Society. *Heart* 1998;80(suppl 2):S1–29.

that our abilities to recognize those who are truly at high risk of coronary disease remain very limited, and that is one of the strongest arguments to change the conventional lipid-based diagnostic system.

(a)

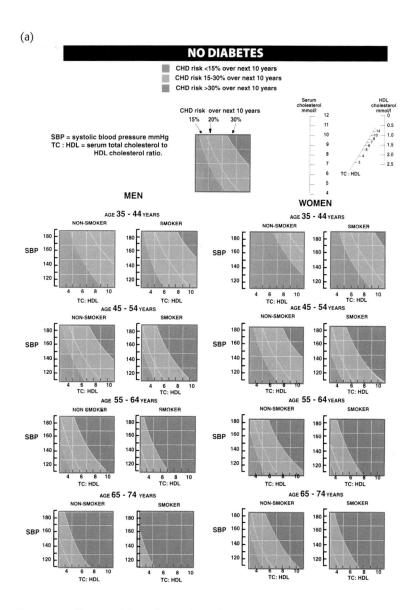

Figure 10.3 Coronary risk prediction charts for men (left) and women (right) without (a) and with (b, opposite) diabetes. The charts should not be used for calculating risk in people with established CHD (previous myocardial infarction and/or angina), with other significant atherosclerosis, left ventricular hypertrophy on ECG, or diabetic patients with proteinuria; these should receive lipid-lowering

(b)

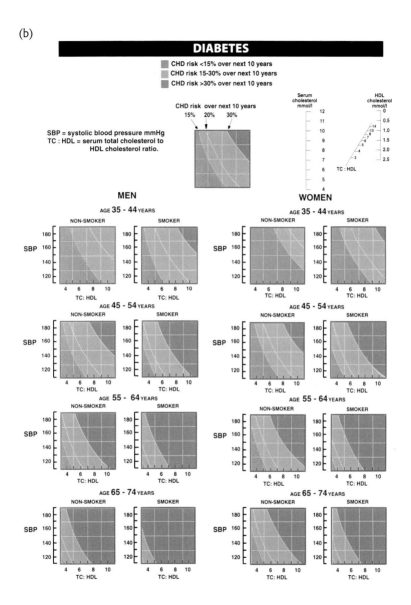

medication in addition to diet modification if their serum cholesterol is 5.0 mmol/L (200 mg/dL) or above. SBP, systolic blood pressure (mmHg); TC:HDL, serum total cholesterol to HDL cholesterol ratio. Reproduced with permission from the University of Manchester, UK.

When to treat – Key points

- Any clinical evidence of vascular disease is an absolute indication to treat. So also is diabetes mellitus in North America.
- Statins are the mainstay of pharmacological therapy.
- Estimation of risk should be broadly based and include age, sex, blood pressure and smoking history as well as lipid levels (and diabetes mellitus in countries where this is not in itself an absolute indication).
- In our opinion, intensive lowering of LDL is the principal objective of therapy.

Key references

Durrington PN, Prais H, Bhatnagar D et al. Indications for the cholesterol-lowering medication: comparison of risk-assessment methods. *Lancet* 1999;353:278–81.

Miremadi S, Sniderman A, Frohlich J. Can measurement of serum apolipoprotein B replace the lipid profile monitoring of patients with lipoprotein disorders? *Clin Chem* 2002;48:484–8.

National Cholesterol Education Program. Executive summary of the third report of the National Cholesterol Education Program (NCEP) Expert Panel on detection, evaluation and treatment of high blood cholesterol in adults (Adult Treatment Panel III). *JAMA* 2001;285:2486–97.

Sniderman AD, Furberg CD, Keech A, Roeters van Lennep JE. Apoproteins versus lipids as indices of coronary risk and as targets for statin therapy: analysis of the evidence. *Lancet*; in press.

Wood D, Durrington PN, Poulter N et al. Joint British Recommendations on prevention of coronary heart disease in clinical practice. *Heart* 1998;80(suppl 2):S1–29.

Non-invasive diagnostic methods for asymptomatic atherosclerosis

These need to be simple, inexpensive and widely available. The electro-cardiogram fulfills all of these criteria and, although it is only rarely helpful in the asymptomatic patient, the test should not be neglected. Bruits in peripheral vessels should be examined with Doppler ultrasound. Treadmill exercise tests are often essential to diagnose chest pain accurately and to determine the ischemic threshold. Echocardiography is not a screening tool to recognize coronary disease, and neither are the more sophisticated stress tests, such as treadmill stress testing, stress echocardiography or radionuclide stress imaging. Coronary calcification scores derived from ultrafast CT scanning have attracted much attention. Just how much they add to the current approach is still not clear, particularly when the expense is taken into account.

Biochemical laboratory tests

Methodological sources of variability. 'Accuracy' describes how closely the results from the particular technique being used in a specific laboratory relate to the results obtained using the accepted reference (or best) method for that variable. That is, how close is the answer in your laboratory to the right answer? All other things being equal, any deviation from the reference method should be systematic. Lack of accuracy or 'bias' makes comparison of results difficult (if not impossible), and therefore the application of guidelines difficult (if not impossible).

'Precision' quantifies the difference in repeated measures of the same sample and is expressed as the coefficient of variation (the standard deviation of the repeated measures divided by their average). That is, how variable would the results from the laboratory be if the same sample were measured repeatedly?

Imprecision and inaccuracy should each be less than 3%. Even within these limits, there can be considerable variance in laboratory reports for the same sample, which is why it is recommended to sample more than once before categorizing lipid levels.

Another criterion to consider is standardization. A test is said to be standardized when all methods that have been approved for routine clinical use yield the same value, because all have been related to an accepted reference. Standardized tests allow results from the same patient, but from different laboratories, to be compared.

Unfortunately, while considerable progress has been made in improving clinical lipid testing, important limitations remain. Only total cholesterol and apoB and apoAI meet all the requirements.

Biological sources of variability are multiple and can be separated into physiological, behavioral and clinical sources of variability.

Age, gender and diet are important modifiers of plasma lipid levels. Clinical factors also need to be taken into account. For example, lipid levels change abruptly and markedly with many illnesses (e.g. myocardial infarction) and operations (e.g. coronary artery bypass surgery), making accurate diagnosis in the acute setting difficult, if not impossible. Serum cholesterol measured within 24 hours of the onset of chest pain in patients with acute myocardial infarction or coronary insufficiency can be a guide to how high the cholesterol was before the acute event. However, it should never be concluded that a level of less than 5.0 mmol/L (200 mg/dL) measured under these circumstances means that statin therapy is unnecessary. In all patients, subsequent levels should be obtained. Certain medications, including steroid sex hormones, can also affect lipid levels (see Chapter 7).

Total cholesterol. Almost all clinical laboratories now use enzymatic techniques to measure cholesterol, and the measurement is rapid, accurate and easily automated. Non-fasting samples can be used. An abnormally high total cholesterol can occasionally be due to either markedly increased HDL cholesterol or chylomicrons. With the latter, depending on the level of triglycerides, the risk of pancreatitis may be augmented.

The virtues of total cholesterol measurement are its simplicity and reliability. The drawbacks are that, with the exception of a small minority with markedly high values, there is little difference between the cholesterol levels of those with and those without coronary disease. Moreover, mild or moderate elevation in LDL cholesterol with concomitant reduction in HDL cholesterol may result in a normal total cholesterol value.

Triglycerides. Enzymatic methods are also the most commonly used means to measure plasma triglycerides. However, these methods are less precise, less accurate and not standardized. Furthermore, as plasma triglycerides rise markedly after a meal due to the entry into plasma of dietary fatty acids such as chylomicron triglycerides, standard practice calls for fasting samples so that generally VLDL triglycerides only will be measured. This imposes considerable difficulty for the patient and considerable uncertainty for the laboratory. However, many patients with coronary disease have impaired chylomicron clearance from plasma after meals, and the increased remnants may contribute to their risk of vascular disease. This feature is difficult to assess in clinical practice if only fasting samples are taken. However, such patients frequently also have an elevated apoB.

LDL cholesterol has become the benchmark laboratory test on which most therapeutic decisions are based. It has many strengths and its value is supported by the epidemiological and therapeutic data gathered over considerable time. Another important advantage is that it is now familiar to many physicians the world over. But it has important limitations, and these should not be overlooked.

First, in most laboratories, it is a calculated value rather than a direct measurement. The usual formulae used are:

$$[\text{LDL cholesterol}] = [\text{total cholesterol}] - \left([\text{HDL cholesterol}] + \left[\frac{\text{triglycerides}}{2.2}\right]\right)$$

if all concentrations are in mmol/L;

$$[\text{LDL cholesterol}] = [\text{total cholesterol}] - \left([\text{HDL cholesterol}] + \left[\frac{\text{triglycerides}}{5}\right]\right)$$

if all concentrations are in mg/dL. Therefore, all the inaccuracies in each test come into play.

Second, it is not standardized and therefore values gained using one method are not necessarily the same as those gained using another, making the application of guidelines somewhat imprecise.

Third, just as with total cholesterol, there is so much overlap in the values of LDL cholesterol between those with and those without coronary disease that, unless levels are markedly elevated or very low, it is of little value in determining risk.

Fourth, LDL cholesterol cannot be calculated when triglycerides are > 4.5 mmol/L (400 mg/dL), and major errors can occur once triglycerides are > 2.0 mmol/L (180 mg/dL).

Fifth, the calculation is also frequently in serious error at target levels of LDL cholesterol, i.e. < 3.0 mmol/L (120 mg/dL).

HDL cholesterol is measured in most clinical laboratories by first precipitating the apoB-containing lipoproteins (VLDL, IDL and LDL) and then measuring cholesterol in the supernatant. There is considerable epidemiological evidence demonstrating that the risk of coronary disease is inversely related to the level of HDL cholesterol. The measurement also has considerable limitations. It is not standardized, and accuracy is particularly critical as there are, in general, only small differences between normal and abnormal levels. Also, it is not clear how a low HDL cholesterol increases the risk of disease. This limitation matters because a low HDL cholesterol frequently coexists with other abnormalities such as a high triglyceride or high apoB value. Furthermore, there is no pharmacological therapy currently available that increases HDL cholesterol only; thus no clinical trials have focused on this effect in isolation.

Ratio of total serum cholesterol to HDL cholesterol. This ratio may provide a better approach; it is, for example, the method used in the charts in Figure 10.3 (see pages 124–5) and includes the risk embodied in LDL cholesterol. There is a wealth of epidemiological data relating to it, and it is therapeutically modifiable by drugs such as statins, albeit because of their effects on LDL cholesterol rather than HDL cholesterol. The ratio also contains in the HDL cholesterol value much of the prognostic information contained in triglyceride values, because these are strongly inversely correlated to HDL. It may therefore have an advantage over serum non-HDL cholesterol (serum cholesterol – HDL cholesterol) values, which have also been proposed as overcoming some of the difficulties posed by indirect estimation of LDL cholesterol.

Apob. Standardized, automated, accurate, inexpensive methods to measure apoB are available. Fasting is not required. There are two forms of apoB: apoB$_{100}$ in VLDL, IDL, LDL and Lp(a), and apoB$_{48}$ in chylomicrons and chylomicron remnants. However, even in the peak postprandial hyperlipidemic state, there so few apoB$_{48}$ particles that fasting is not required. Furthermore, even in hypertriglyceridemic subjects, more than 90% of the total apoB particles are LDL particles and therefore total plasma apoB is really determined by LDL apoB.

ApoAI is one of the major apolipoproteins in HDL and can also be accurately and precisely measured using standardized automated assays. There is an inverse correlation with risk as with HDL cholesterol. The two are likely equivalent with regard to categorization of risk.

Apob:apoAI ratio is the apolipoprotein equivalent of the total:HDL cholesterol ratio. The AMORIS study has shown the apoB/apoA1 to be superior to total/HDL cholesterol as a summary index of the risk of vascular disease.

Lp(a). For now, Lp(a) can only be measured in a few laboratories. Considerable work remains to be done in standardizing the assay before it can be broadly introduced into clinical practice (see page 133).

Clinical and laboratory tests – Key points

- LDL cholesterol is calculated, not measured, and there are important limitations on its accuracy. Fasting samples are essential.
- Measurement of ApoB and apoAI is standardized, and values can be determined on non-fasting samples.
- The ratios apoB/apoAI and total cholesterol / HDL cholesterol express the overall risk of disease due to dyslipoproteinemia. The ratio of the apolipoproteins is even more precise than the ratio of the lipids.

Key reference

Rifai N, Warnick GR, Dominiczak MH, eds. *Handbook of Lipoprotein Testing*, 2nd edn. Washington: American Association for Clinical Chemistry Press, 2000.

Clinical measurements

Apob. Given that apoB measurement has been standardized and it is neither difficult nor expensive to perform, it should be possible to overcome the arguments against its introduction as a routine test.

Small, dense LDL increases the risk of vascular disease. As increased LDL particle number and small, dense LDL often coexist, it has been difficult to be sure of the degree of risk conferred by the small, dense LDL. However, the Quebec Cardiovascular Study has demonstrated that an elevated apoB doubles the risk of coronary disease and small, dense LDL increases the risk six-fold. There are no routine methods currently available for the detection of small, dense LDL. However, a plasma triglyceride level over 1.5 mmol/L (140 mg/dL) should raise suspicion of the presence of small, dense LDL.

Lp(a) is present in serum, and shows considerable interindividual variation. Its level is related to CHD and stroke risk. It is greatly increased in patients with any type of renal disease and in many patients with FH. Lp(a) measurement is not currently available for routine patient evaluation. It may, however, assume greater importance if a safe and effective therapeutic approach to lowering Lp(a) appears and is shown to decrease the incidence of vascular disease. The measurement of Lp(a) will have to be improved, as the marked variations in its composition and molecular weight make comparison among individuals more difficult than is usually recognized.

Plasma homocysteine. Much interest has been generated by recent studies linking increased risk of vascular disease to increased plasma homocysteine levels. However, until clinical trial evidence and its routine measurement become available, it will be impossible to incorporate homocysteine into routine clinical practice. Physicians will have to continue to use their clinical judgment as to whether folate supplementation should be given to patients with vascular disease.

Plasma fibrinogen and plasminogen activator inhibitor increases have also been linked to increased risk. More information is needed on how much their measurement adds to risk assessment, particularly after other risk factors are included in the evaluation. Overall, however, any final strategy of risk assessment will ideally include a thorough evaluation of a range of prothrombogenic factors.

New methods to diagnose presymptomatic vascular disease
This is the area in which the greatest progress should be made. Methods are needed to identify early non-occlusive vascular disease. At the moment, carotid ultrasound is helpful, at least with respect to moderate lesions. Unfortunately, at present, the technique is too operator-dependent and too expensive to be widely available. At least the proximal portions of the coronary arteries can be visualized by transesophageal echocardiography, but this will never be a practical general screening method. Ultrafast computed tomography can detect coronary calcification, and this relates at least in a general way to the extent of coronary disease. The method is non-invasive but may not be sufficiently selective to be of practical value. Magnetic resonance imaging of the coronary arteries holds great promise, but expense may unfortunately limit its widespread use.

Clinical trials
The first-generation clinical trials of primary and secondary prevention showed that LDL lowering reduced clinical events without significant side-effects. But they do not define the therapeutic targets. There are other important objectives for clinical trials. Are triglyceride-lowering agents effective and if so what is the mechanism responsible? Does combination therapy add to clinical benefit? We must also acknowledge that we lack definitive knowledge about the value of lipid-lowering therapy in critical subgroups. At least numerically, people with diabetes may make up the largest group. The initial trials suggest substantial benefit from LDL lowering. However, the lipid profiles of the diabetics

in these trials are not typically encountered, and subgroup analyses do not substitute for a primary test of the hypothesis.

All in all, there is much still to be learnt about hyperlipidemia and its role in disease prevention. Moreover, there is a great deal that still needs to be done in clinical practice to take full advantage of what is already known. An important and realizable objective for the immediate future is to implement fully the conclusions of our existing knowledge of the treatment of hyperlipidemia.

Future trends – Key points

- Apolipoprotein measurement should be available in routine clinical practice.
- With further development, tissue-based diagnosis by ultrasound, or by ultrafast CT and MRI, might offer considerable help in early diagnosis so long as their costs can be contained.

Key references

Danesh J, Collins R, Peto R. Lipoprotein (a) and coronary heart disease: meta-analysis of prospective studies. *Circulation* 2000;102:1082–5.

Suckling K, Fears R. Future developments in drug therapy. In: Betteridge DJ et al., eds. *Lipoproteins in Health and Disease*. London: Arnold, 1999:1267–77.

Useful addresses

American Diabetes Association
ATTN: Customer Service,
1701 North Beauregard Street,
Alexandria, VA 22311, USA
phone: 1 800 342 2383
www.diabetes.org

British Heart Foundation
14 Fitzhardinge Street,
London W1H 4DH, UK
phone: 020 7935 0185
fax: 020 7486 5820
internet@bhf.org.uk

Canadian Cardiovascular Society
CCS Secretariat,
222 Queen Street, Suite 1403,
Ottawa, Ontario K1P 5V9,
Canada
phone: 613 569 3407
fax: 613 569 6574
ccsinfo@ccs.ca
www.ccs.ca/

Diabetes UK (DUK)
10 Parkway, London NW1 7AA,
UK
phone: 020 7424 1000
fax: 020 7424 1001
info@diabetes.org.uk

European Atherosclerosis Society
(EAS)
EAS Secretariat:
Professor Sebastiano Calandra,
Sezione di Patologia Generale,

Dipartimento di Scienze
Biomediche,
Universita di Modena e Reggio
Emilia,
Via Campi 287, I-41100 Modena,
Italy
phone: +39 059 2055 423/4116
fax: +39 059 2055 426
sebcal@unimo.it

European Association for the Study
of Diabetes (EASD)
Rheindorfer Weg 3, D-40591,
Düsseldorf, Germany
phone: +49 211 7584690
fax: +49 211 75846929
easd@uni-duesseldorf.de

Hyperlipidemia Education and
Research Trust (HEART) UK
7 North Road, Maidenhead,
Berkshire SL6 1PL, UK
phone: 01628 628638
fax: 01628 628 698
fh@familyheart.org

National Cholesterol Education
Program (NCEP)
www.nhlbi.nih.gov/about/ncep/
index.htm

NCEP Clinical Practice Guidelines for
Cholesterol Management in Adults
(ATPIII)
www.nhlbi.nih.gov/guidelines/
cholesterol/index.htm

Index